Hypnosis

Communicate to Your Inner Self and to Control Your Destiny

(The Technique to Hypnotize Yourself Into Hypnotic Realities)

Michael Whitely

Published By **Neal David**

Michael Whitely

Hypnosis: Communicate to Your Inner Self and to Control Your Destiny (The Technique to Hypnotize Yourself Into Hypnotic Realities)

ISBN 978-1-7751139-9-7

Legal & Disclaimer

The information contained in this book is not designed to replace or take the place of any form of medicine or professional medical advice. The information in this book has been provided for educational & entertainment purposes only.

The information contained in this book has been compiled from sources deemed reliable, and it is accurate to the best of the Author's knowledge; however, the Author cannot guarantee its accuracy and validity and cannot be held liable for any errors or omissions. Changes are periodically made to this book. You must consult your doctor or get professional medical advice before using any of the suggested remedies, techniques, or information in this book.

Upon using the information contained in this book, you agree to hold harmless the Author from and against any damages, costs, and expenses, including any legal fees potentially resulting from the application of any of the information provided by this guide. This disclaimer applies to any damages or injury caused by the use and application, whether directly or indirectly, of any advice or information presented, whether for breach of contract, tort, negligence, personal injury, criminal intent, or under any other cause of action.

You agree to accept all risks of using the information presented inside this book. You need to consult a professional medical practitioner in order to ensure you are both able and healthy enough to participate in this program.

Table Of Contents

Chapter 1: The Truth about Rapid Hypnosis

Have you ever heard the announcing "the mind is extra powerful than you accept as true with you studied"? Of route you have got were given. But have you ever in reality had a 2d to stop and don't forget the proper quantity of that electricity? As you're taking a seat there, reading these words, your thoughts are in a country of consistent activity. Every idea, every emotion, each belief has an effect on the way you experience the area around you.

But proper right here comes the real query: Are you on pinnacle of factors of that power? Or as an alternative, do you revel in that the energy is on top of things of you?

We live in an technology of misinformation, in which hypnosis, in particular, has been the sufferer of misunderstandings, Hollywood exaggerations and famous myths. Ever because of the truth I have turn out to be a little one, I become inquisitive about the ones TV suggests wherein the hypnotist snapped his arms and those, as though they had been zombies, decided his orders. However, the truth is a lot extra charming and masses lots much less dramatic.

So why is that this subject matter so critical? Because the energy of rapid hypnosis has the capability to unencumbered that awesome internal ability that often lies dormant because of proscribing beliefs and deceptive myths. What if I knowledgeable you that, in choice to being a TV show, hypnosis is a tool you can use to convert your lifestyles, get proper of access to internal resources and acquire dreams you in no way imagined feasible?

Hypnosis isn't magic, despite the fact that it may enjoy magical. It is a shape of verbal exchange with that inner maximum and maximum powerful part of your being: the subconscious. It is that place wherein your ideals, memories, habits and automated responses that lead you to behave in a single manner or a few other are residing.

But in advance than we dive right in, permit me ask you a question. Think of a time at the identical time as your mind executed a trick on you. Have you ever located your self in a situation in which you knew you have to not do some factor, however ended up doing it besides? Like the ones chocolates you promised yourself you wouldn't devour but ended up mysteriously disappearing from the fridge.

That, my friend, is your unconscious in motion.

This economic spoil seeks to get to the lowest of and demystify what rapid hypnosis simply is. What you can discover also can marvel you. You might also even question what you generally perception you knew approximately your personal mind. But I promise you that, with the useful resource of the end of this adventure, you'll be armed with effective and realistic understanding.

You may be questioning, "Wait! If this emerge as so effective, why is not all of us using it?" Well, it is because of the truth, as with many powerful topics, fear and lack of knowledge have woven a veil of thriller round it.

In the following few pages, we're able to begin to carry that veil. With an open and willing thoughts, I invite you to embark on this revealing adventure to discover the reality approximately rapid hypnosis, and the way it can be your best friend in conquering your best dreams and desires.

So, are you organized for a deep journey into the depths of your thoughts? Ready to break a long way from vintage notions and encompass a state-of-the-art information that empowers you? If the solution is positive, look at on. Because this journey has certainly all began out.

And as soon as I say "adventure", I am not talking approximately surely any adventure, but one that has been traveled through many, in the route of records, searching out solutions about the real capacity of the human thoughts. Ancient philosophers, which includes Plato, already confused about the nature of truth and the way our belief may be fashioned. However, it modified into James Braid in 1843, who coined the time period "hypnosis", derived from the Greek term "hypnos", which means that that dream.

But, in spite of the fact that the time period suggests "sleep," hypnosis isn't a country of drowsiness. Rather, it's far a nation of acute awareness. Dr. Milton Erickson, one of the most influential hypnotherapists of the twentieth century and creator of Hypnotherapy: An Innovative Approach (1973), argued that all people enjoy hypnotic states in our each day lives. Have you ever turn out to be so immersed in a ebook or film which you misplaced tune of the time and place round you? That, high-priced reader, is a trance u.S.A., much like that finished with hypnosis.

Now, you may ask, "If hypnosis is surely a rustic of awareness, how can it have plenty electricity?" Well, it is simple. In this nation, our subconscious mind becomes pretty liable to new mind and pointers. Imagine your mind as a garden. In the normal us of a, that garden has a excessive fence, shielding it. But in a hypnotic country, that fence disappears, permitting new seeds to be planted.

The renowned clinical psychologist, Dr. Brian Alman, in his paintings Self-Hypnosis for Personal Achievement (1991), states that thru hypnosis, not remarkable can we plant new seeds, however we also can dispose of weeds, i.E., poor beliefs and conduct that prevent us from moving in advance.

Now, it's far vital to emphasise that, despite the fact that hypnosis may be effective, it isn't a magic wand. You cannot virtually hypnotize your self and anticipate all of your problems to disappear. It is a tool that, used well, can beautify your private increase and development.

That said, over time, there was a few resistance to the idea of hypnosis. Thanks to exaggerated portrayals in films and television suggests, many human beings bear in mind that hypnosis is a few shape of thoughts manage, wherein one may be pressured to act towards their will. This could not be similarly from the truth. Hypnosis is a nation of cooperation a number of the hypnotist and the hassle.

Now, as you take a look at on, I want you to expect a global wherein you could communicate proper away collectively together together with your subconscious, wherein you may have an impact on your ideals and behavior for the better. A international in which your mind, this is already fairly powerful, will become even more effective.

Wouldn't that be wonderful?

As we circulate similarly into this financial ruin, I invite you to allow cross of any skepticism or doubt and include the opportunity of what is to go back.

Because, as the famous hypnotherapist Dave Elman stated in Hypnotherapy (1964), "The mind is the vital thing that opens the door to limitless possibilities." And with each word you check, you've got become towards that door.

The extraordinary Nadia Comăneci, the Romanian gymnast who bowled over the world on the 1976 Montreal Olympics, confessed in her autobiography, Letters to a Young Gymnast (2003), that she used visualization and hypnosis strategies to rehearse her workouts mentally. Before each fashionable overall performance, she discovered herself executing every movement with perfection, feeling the experience of feat even in advance than she jumped on degree.

But it isn't always fine in the sports sports region wherein hypnosis has showed to be contemporary. Imagine an man or woman who has smoked for two decades and has attempted infinite instances to kick the dependancy with out success. With the help of hypnosis, and through specific tips, that character can start to see smoking from a totally exceptional attitude, perceiving it as a few factor remote places and a long way off. Richard Bandler, co-founder of Neurolinguistic Programming and creator of Essential Transformation (1985), has documented more than one cases of humans who have give up smoking, reduced their tension, or overcome phobias in report time via hypnotic techniques.

But what makes hypnosis so effective in the ones cases? Dr. Michael Yapko, in Trancework: A Comprehensive Approach to Hypnosis (2003), indicates that hypnosis works precisely as it lets in us to get entry to our middle ideals and values. Instead of searching for to fight our behavior and behaviors from the outside, hypnosis lets in us to trade them from the internal. It is like having direct get right of get entry to to to the software software software of our thoughts and being capable of beautify it to an stepped forward model of ourselves.

Now, I'd which include you to perform a little mental exercising. Imagine for a 2nd a place of your existence that you would love to beautify. It can be your health, your profession, your relationships... Something. Now, undergo in mind which you have the electricity to speak at once to that part of you that controls that vicinity. Imagine that you may educate it, encourage it, and align it collectively collectively together with your private desires. Feel the exhilaration and revel in of control that might provide you with.

Surprising, isn't it?

But right here comes the honestly exciting component. The exercise you without a doubt did is a shape of hypnosis. It is a sample of what you can obtain by means of connecting at the side of your mind at a deeper degree. Because, at the surrender of the day, hypnosis isn't always something extra than verbal exchange: communication with the simplest and often most forgotten part of ourselves.

And as you still glide in advance on this journey of discovery, allow me to percent with you a quote from the prominent Carl Jung, who in his paintings The Psychology of Transference (1946) wrote: "Until you are making the subconscious conscious, it's going to direct your existence and you will call it future". I invite you to mirror on those phrases as you put together for the subsequent segment of our journey together. For, steeply-priced reader, what follows is truly transformative.

Chapter 2: The Hidden Key to Your Inner Power

Think approximately the very last time you surprised yourself, whether or not it changed into with a sudden burst of creativity, an resourceful method to a trouble that turned into plaguing you, or possibly in truth on the same time as you remembered the name of someone you hadn't visible for years. Have you ever perplexed wherein that energy comes from?

You do no longer need to look far. The answer lies right inside the again of your eyes, pulsing and pulsating with an almost electric powered powered powered strength. It's your mind, a form that, with its about 86 billion neurons, resembles a miniature universe, packed with interconnected stars.

But why is the brain so essential in our discussion of hypnosis? The solution is simple: because of the fact every hypnotic method, whether or not or now not self-imposed or guided by using way of some one of a kind, has its primary setting on this organ. Understanding the way it really works is essential to unlocking your inner strength and using hypnosis as a device for transformation.

Now, believe for a 2nd that you can have direct get entry to to each corner of your brain, that you could turn advantageous regions on or off at will, and that you may software application or reprogram any feature or dependancy you desired. Sounds tempting, does no longer it? That is exactly what hypnosis allows you to do. But in advance than we delve into the wonders of this historical artwork, it's far crucial that we have a look at a chunk extra about nature's maximum state-of-the-art device: our thoughts.

Oliver Sacks, in his work "The Man Who Mistook His Wife for a Hat" (1985), gave us a panoramic view of strategies the smallest anomalies within the mind can create exchange worlds and realities. If the easy displacement of a neuron may want to have such consequences, bear in mind what we have to obtain if we discovered out to direct and channel the electricity and capability of our mind.

In this financial ruin, I promise that not handiest will you get to recognize your thoughts in a manner you in no manner imagined earlier than, but in the long run, you'll be amazed at how an awful lot electricity you have got were given been carrying spherical with you all along that, until now, has remained hidden. The technology within the again of hypnosis is deeper than it appears within the starting appearance. But as we plunge into the depths of our being, we emerge with renewed power and readability.

Are you equipped for this adventure, prepared to unfastened up secrets and techniques and techniques and strategies that have been locked for your mind for years, perhaps a few years? As you study, I invite you to keep an open mind, to question, to reflect and, surely, to count on. Because the journey for your internal strength isn't always simplest a smooth analyzing; it is a transformative revel in.

In fact, this complete way of self-exploration and discovery isn't always new. Throughout records, humanity has sought techniques to recognize and, if feasible, control the talents and talents of its mind. Meditation, yoga and distinct age-vintage practices, in essence, have this equal reason. But hypnosis, specially, has verified to be a sincerely effective tool in this quest.

If we look again to 1890, William James, in his paintings "Principles of Psychology", knowledgeable us about the plasticity of the human thoughts, that precise ability to conform, analyze and evolve. Although he did not have the technological tool we have have been given nowadays, he understood a critical reality: that the mind is malleable. And if it's miles malleable, it's miles influenceable. This is wherein hypnosis comes into play.

Tell me, have you ever ever been so immersed in an hobby or concept that the outdoor worldwide appears to vanish away? That extreme hobby, that state of waft, is a shape of trance. And in that trance, your mind is jogging at best stages, growing connections, solidifying ideas and, regularly, organising as lots as new opportunities.

Norman Doidge, in "The Brain That Heals Itself" (2007), confirmed us extraordinary testimonies of folks who, in competition to all odds, overcame thoughts obstacles manner to the thoughts's capability to rewire itself. Now, remember combining that inherent capability of the thoughts with the strength of hypnosis. The possibilities are actually countless.

So what exactly takes vicinity at some stage in hypnosis? In essence, you're getting access to an altered kingdom of reputation, a country in which your unconscious mind becomes more receptive. While your aware mind analyzes, judges and criticizes, your unconscious thoughts accepts and acts. And it is on this incredible and mysterious realm of the unconscious that your real strength is dwelling. It is proper right here that you can reprogram beliefs, conquer boundaries and unharness your proper functionality.

Remember that antique adage that we most effective use 10% of our mind? Although scientifically that determine is a myth, what's proper is that maximum human beings not regularly get proper of access to or make use of the vastness of property and skills that our mind has to offer. Hypnosis, on this sense, is the key that unlocks that special ninety% (metaphorically speaking).

So, are you prepared to dive deeper? Ready to resolve greater secrets and techniques and techniques which have been patiently ready to be located? Let's hold going, because of the reality this journey is a long manner from over. A global of wonder and discovery awaits us. I guarantee you that, with every internet web page you turn, you could get in the direction of that version of your self which you continually knew existed, but possibly in no manner knew the manner to attain.

The strength of the mind is terrific, is not it? But come on, permit me let you know a story that illustrates exactly how profound this power can be.

Imagine Elena, a professional pianist who spent a wonderful deal of her life immersed in tune. At the age of 30, an twist of future took away the mobility of her right hand. Doctors cautioned her she ought to by no means play the piano the same manner once more. But as opposed to accepting this assessment, Elena decided to take control. She began the use of hypnosis to visualise her hand shifting with the same dexterity and talent as before. Every day, she could pass into a deep trance and "exercising" in her mind, feeling each keystroke and each movement. And some aspect fantastic befell: over the years, and toward all scientific odds, he started out out to regain motion in his hand.

This instance is not an remoted case. Oliver Sacks, in "The Man Who Mistook His Wife for a Hat" (1985), relates reminiscences of patients with neurological troubles who found unusual and regularly sudden tactics to conform and overcome their conditions. While the ones instances did no longer usually comprise hypnosis, they did display the brain's outstanding potential to conform, alternate, and heal.

These aren't mere miracles. They are testaments to the big strength of our mind and what it can accomplish at the same time as we direct it with purpose and motive. Through hypnosis, we are capable of get proper of access to that a part of the thoughts this is moldable, that learns, adapts and overcomes limitations.

But, of path, you'll be asking your self, "Would this honestly paintings for me?" And it's a legitimate question. However, maintain in thoughts this: each and each one people has skilled a few shape of self-hypnosis in our lives, despite the fact that we did not realize it. Have you ever been so immersed in a e-book that the arena spherical you appears to vanish? Or have you ever driven domestic and, even as you arrive, you do no longer precisely undergo in mind the electricity? These are examples of moderate trance, altered states of cognizance that every person enjoy glaringly.

So what takes place at the same time as we take manage of these states and direct them inside the direction of a particular purpose? The answer is simple: transformation.

Let's do a highbrow exercise now, we must? Imagine a door in the the front of you. This door represents the get right of entry to to those unexplored areas of your mind. Now, recollect you have got were given a golden key on your hand, the critical factor of hypnosis. As you turn it, the door slowly opens, revealing a international of infinite opportunities. Would you dare to enter?

But, allow's get another time to fact for a second and preserve digging. What do specialists say approximately the hidden capacity of our mind and the way hypnosis can launch it? Let's check it inside the subsequent segment. I promise it's going to take you inside the route of the vital element which could launch your internal energy.

The journey via the recesses of our mind is as giant because the universe itself. Every belief, every emotion and every memory are stars shining inside the darkish sky of our unconscious. And as we find out this huge cosmos, we encounter an irrefutable truth: the thoughts is without a doubt the command middle, the seat of our identification, the reason force of our human experience.

According to Norman Doidge, in his artwork "The Brain That Changes Itself" (2007), neuroplasticity suggests us that our thoughts cells, or neurons, can reconfigure themselves based totally on our reviews. This capacity to evolve is what permits individuals like Elena, the pianist, to get better in competition to all odds. But what if we have to deliberately beautify this adaptability? What if we should, thru hypnosis, consciously direct this technique?

For a 2nd, endure in thoughts the outcomes. You can also need to conquer vintage traumas, eliminate harmful conduct, collect capabilities at an extended tempo and lots extra. If the mind is a laptop, then hypnosis is the software software program that permits us to reprogram and optimize our operation.

Chapter 3: Preparing the Mind for Hypnosis

Have you ever tried to check a very new know-how? Perhaps you don't forget the initial feeling of awkwardness, the hesitation, the doubt. Now, trust that as opposed to reading to play a musical instrument or have a study a latest language, you got down to get right of entry to the vastness of your mind's energy. Sounds daunting, does not it? And yet, the proper steerage can turn that mountain into an thrilling and possible route.

Why is it critical to put together the mind for hypnosis? Well, preserve in thoughts hypnosis as a journey. Imagine you are about to embark on a cruise on the ocean of your subconscious. You do not set sail on a supply with out ensuring the whole thing is in region, proper? Similarly, intellectual schooling guarantees that your hypnosis adventure is straightforward, powerful and, specially, transformative.

Now, as you technique that, go through in mind this: How may additionally need to you sense if I counseled you that this training isn't best vital however additionally distinctly easy? It could probable appear to be a contradiction, but because the high-quality author F. Scott Fitzgerald stated in "The Great Gatsby" (1925), "The take a look at of a awesome intelligence is the capacity to keep opposing thoughts in mind at the identical time and however preserve the capability to characteristic." In this example, energy and ease can coexist in concord.

Hypnosis, opposite to well-known fable, is not a mysterious, esoteric altered united states that only a select out few can get right of access to. In fact, anybody experience hypnotic states several times an afternoon. Have you ever been out of region in concept whilst searching out the window? Or have you pushed domestic and barely remembered the pressure? These are natural trance states that anybody experience.

Seizing those moments and getting prepared your thoughts for a deeper hypnotic experience is an paintings in itself. But how do you do it?

Here's a query to ponder: What makes an enjoy memorable? Is it the surroundings? The people involved? Or is it the dominion of thoughts you are in? As you immerse yourself inside the ones reflections, you may begin to apprehend that the actual adventure of hypnosis starts offevolved extended earlier than you are taking a seat in a chair or pay interest a mild voice guiding you right into a country of relaxation. The actual magic starts offevolved inside you, inside the manner you put together yourself for the revel in.

Talking about making prepared the mind can also seem like an precis concept, but in reality it is a tangible, measurable and, most importantly, plausible manner. Therefore, as you embark in this economic disaster, I invite you to open your self to the possibility of coming across the manner to prepare your thoughts, no longer simplest for hypnosis, however for any new mastering or enjoy to your existence.

In short, making organized your thoughts is like tuning an device. And, if you do it successfully, the following tune is a symphony of limitless opportunities. Are you prepared to analyze the manner? Of route you are. After all, you've come this a protracted way with reason and backbone. So take a deep breath and prepare to immerse yourself in the marvel of self-discovery. Because the real adventure, my pricey reader, is just beginning.

Since you have already understood the significance of having geared up your mind for hypnosis, you can assume that the following step is actually to dive right in. However, endure in thoughts for a 2d Sun Tzu's philosophy in "The Art of War" (circa 5th century B.C.): "The war is received earlier than it's far fought." Thus, it is clever to recognize that proper education and a strong foundation need to make the difference amongst an ephemeral hypnotic enjoy and a simply transformative one.

As we delve deeper into this coaching, we come upon severa assets that have addressed the task of the mind and its strength. Carl Jung, in his paintings "Psychological Types" (1921), stated the thoughts as a giant ocean wherein our aware thoughts are only the top of the iceberg, while most of our being is living deep within the unconscious. To get proper of entry to this intensity, education is pinnacle. But how can we put together ourselves?

Knowledge: Often worry and resistance come from lack of expertise. Understanding what hypnosis is, the way it truly works and what its benefits are, will allow you to technique it with an open mind.

Environment: Imagine looking for to meditate within the middle of a noisy birthday party. Difficult, isn't it? In the identical way, hypnosis requires a appropriate surroundings: quiet, freed from distractions, and wherein you sense safe and snug.

Intention: The mind is strong, and as such, the aim you location in the again of any motion performs a vital feature. Why do you want to exercising hypnosis? What do you desire to benefit? Being clean about your why offers you motive and focuses your mind.

Practice: Like any potential, hypnosis improves with exercising. Don't count on to be a draw close on your first try. Give your thoughts time and patience to conform and have a look at.

In fact, Aldous Huxley in "The Doors of Perception" (1954) proposed the concept that our thoughts is kind of a filter out, and that hypnosis, meditation and extraordinary strategies can help "open" this clear out to allow us to get right of access to greater notion and focus.

You may be asking your self, "Do I really need all this education? Can't I truely strive?" And the answer is: of direction you could. But isn't always it better to provide your mind the first-class possible threat of fulfillment?

as you go through this adventure, I encourage you to remember Aristotle's terms: "We are what we repeatedly do. Therefore, excellence is not an act, however a dependancy." With proper education, you are cultivating the addiction of excellence in hypnosis, permitting you to discover and harness the top notch power of your thoughts. Are you organized to preserve to delve into this interesting worldwide? Of direction you are. Because every step you are taking brings you towards coming across the proper strength that is residing internal you.

Going deeper into the heart of the steerage, we do not forget that, at some stage, we've all experienced altered states of popularity. Perhaps within the ones moments virtually in advance than you fall asleep, wherein fact seems blurred, or even as you lose your self in a ebook and time seems to fly. These states are natural and, in fact, much like hypnosis.

Now, have you ever ever considered how a good deal language influences our notion of truth? Ludwig Wittgenstein, in "Philosophical Investigations" (1953), said: "The limits of my language are the boundaries of my global". Words have power, and inside the international of hypnosis, this strength is magnified.

Imagine for a moment a lush forest, wherein every tree represents a notion or concept you preserve. Some bushes are antique and robust, deeply rooted on your thoughts. Others are more youthful shoots, smooth, new thoughts which can be virtually beginning to take root. Now, consider that hypnosis is sort of a pathway that lets in you to move among the ones wooden, understand them, and if important, regulate them. Language is the automobile that permits this motion.

Let's have a have a take a look at a concrete instance. Suppose you have got a worry of public talking and this belief is cemented for your thoughts with the useful aid of a past enjoy. Through hypnosis, you may discover that memory, apprehend it and, extra importantly, redefine it. Instead of recalling that moment with tension, you may remodel it proper into a deliver of energy, remembering the way you overcame that second and how it has made you more potent. Hypnotic language helps this alteration, permitting you to speak without delay in your unconscious.

Erik Erikson, in his paintings "Childhood and Society" (1950), referred to identity crises and how they'll be an critical a part of our development. Through hypnosis, you could face and resolve the ones crises, redefining who you are and the way you notice your self.

However, there may be one detail we cannot ignore: trust. Hypnosis calls for self notion, both within the machine and in your self. If you constantly doubt whether or not "this may artwork" or "it's far honestly for you," you are installing location obstacles in your thoughts. On the alternative hand, if you method it with an open mind, trusting the method and your capability to change and boom, the sky's the limit.

Of course, you'll be thinking if there is any guarantee that hypnosis will art work. Well, is there any guarantee in existence that something works? What there is is evidence, studies and testimonials from humans who have converted their lives through hypnosis. But on the prevent of the day, the actual figuring out detail is you.

So, as we keep this adventure, I inspire you to agree with, to consider and to open yourself to the endless possibilities your mind offers you. Because, as Carl Jung as quickly as stated, "Until you are making the unconscious aware, it will run your life and you could name it destiny."

Now that we've got were given explored the depth of the thoughts and the resonance of language, it's miles crucial to apprehend that hypnosis is an paintings as an entire lot as it is a science. And like numerous artwork, practice, staying electricity and passion are important to understand it.

The legendary creator and psychologist, William James, in his traditional "Principles of Psychology" (1890), said: "The finest discovery of my era is that a man or woman can change his life through changing his highbrow thoughts-set". This idea is the center of hypnosis. By enhancing your highbrow mind-set, you may release doors on your thoughts that you may no longer in reality have regarded existed.

Take, as an instance, the idea of autosuggestion. Emile Coué, famous for his autosuggestion method, regularly stated, "Every day, in every manner, I am getting better and better." Although it is able to sound like a easy announcement, it is, in essence, a hypnosis device. Repeating it, believing it and residing it may result in awesome adjustments for your existence.

Have you ever puzzled why a few people have unwavering self-control at the same time as others constantly warfare? An essential part of the solution lies in how they speak with themselves, how they use language to shape their fact.

There are instances, of path, at the same time as you can enjoy skeptical. "Can some factor as smooth as converting the manner I communicate or assume in reality make a distinction?" you may ask. The answer is a powerful positive. Think about it: if a clean exchange in diet plan can remodel a body, why couldn't a change in questioning redesign a thoughts?

And with that in mind, permit me provide you with a piece preview of what's to come back back. Are you prepared to find out the real energy of terms? In the following financial disaster, we're going to get to the bottom of the subtleties of language, from how a smooth word can incite an emotion to how a properly-established sentence can change a destiny. We'll discover collectively the manner to use language to create effective recommendations, capable of generating right away success.

So, are you prepared to keep? Because if there can be one issue for sure, it's miles that this adventure has simply started out.

I promise that thru the prevent of this journey, you cannot great understand the power of hypnosis, however you may moreover have the machine to rouse your internal energy. The subsequent web page is asking ahead to you. Don't leave it prepared.

Chapter 4: The Power of Words

Have you ever felt the power that runs down your backbone even as you pay interest powerful phrases or phrases? Have you located how your day can take a 100 eighty-degree turn definitely due to the fact someone says a few thing that makes you vibrate inner? And the fact is, steeply-priced reader, phrases aren't truely easy combos of letters; they may be keys which could open doorways to new realities.

Now, you can ask, why do phrases have a lot energy? Give that question a 2nd. Allow it to resonate on your mind. Let it settle in and absorb its essence.

Words have the strength to assemble and destroy. They have been the tool of extremely good leaders to unite worldwide places, encourage movements and alternate data. On the opportunity hand, they have got additionally been gadget of manipulation, triggering wars and causing despair. As Rudyard Kipling said in 1923, "Words are, of route, the most effective drug used by mankind." And he couldn't be extra right.

Within hypnosis, this electricity is magnified exponentially. Through a cautious and planned choice of words, you could suggest, guide or maybe dictate a particular final consequences inside the thoughts of the listener. Imagine having that key that unlocks doors in the thoughts, allowing you to get right of access to resources, talents and feelings you did now not even understand you had. It's magical, is not it?

Dr. Milton Erickson (1901-1980), extensively considered the daddy of present day hypnotherapy, understood this energy profoundly. In his studies and medical paintings, he tested that the proper phrases, brought on the proper time and with the proper aim, can bring about amazing states of trance, recovery and transformation.

Here's the trick: it is no longer simply what you are saying, however the way you say it. Tone, rhythm and, of route, phrase preference play important roles. Have you ever sat thru a crackling fireplace, feeling the warmth on your pores and pores and skin, being attentive to the crackling of the flames and dropping your self within the hypnotic dance of the fireside? That sensation, that deep connection to the prevailing second, is what we goal for with language in hypnosis.

Now, steeply-priced reader, as you immerse your self on this monetary disaster, I challenge you to open your mind. To allow these words manual you, not great on a journey of reading, but furthermore on a journey into your very personal inner strength. Because, in spite of everything, isn't always that the factor of this e-book? As you have a look at along, you may come to apprehend that there may be honestly more power to your terms than you ever imagined.

But, if you're nonetheless skeptical, stick round! There is lots greater to discover, and I promise that every internet web page will supply you closer to that revelation. Because, at the forestall of the day, words are truly the begin. There is a whole universe inner you prepared to be explored, and those pages, luxurious reader, are your superstar map.

So take a deep breath, loosen up and allow yourself be carried away with the useful resource of the go together with the flow of phrases and mind that lets in you to present themselves. And as you achieve this, usually do not forget the immortal word of the poet Edward Bulwer-Lytton (1803-1873): "The pen is mightier than the sword". In the context of hypnosis, we could say that "the phrase is mightier than each different tool".

With that, we flip to the coronary heart of our problem rely. Are you equipped to find out the actual electricity of words and the way they may be your top notch friend on the journey to at once fulfillment? Go ahead! Because, in the long run, the energy is already internal you. It's time to discover ways to unleash it.

Language, if used effectively, becomes as powerful a device as a chisel inside the fingers of a sculptor. With every phrase, with every phrase, we sculpt the truth we desire. In the arena of hypnosis, the electricity of the word takes on a deeper which means that, and it is proper right here that the paintings of fantastic authors will become a essential pillar.

Richard Bandler and John Grinder of their paintings "The Structure of Magic" (1975) provided us with a awesome perception into how phrases carry together our truth. They argued that our language no longer simplest describes truth, but creates it. What we're announcing, how we're pronouncing it, and the phrases we select are reflections of our inner representation of the area. But what if we may additionally moreover want to adjust that illustration sincerely with the aid of way of fixing our language?

Let's recollect a hypothetical scenario. Imagine you are a shop clerk and you're faced with an not sure purchaser. Instead of announcing, "Would you want to shop for this?", you could rephrase and say, "How heaps should you want to revel in the advantages of this product?". Notice the distinction, you're not selling a product; you are selling an enjoy, a benefit. You've changed the focus of the communique, and with it, the consumer's mindset.

This technique, known as "reframing" or rephrasing, is simply one of the many device we're capable of draw from the sector of hypnosis and NLP (Neuro Linguistic Programming). The idea is simple: change the way you communicate about something, and you can trade the manner you reflect onconsideration on it.

However, it isn't simplest the form of the phrases that topics, but the tone and context. Stephen R. Covey in "The 7 Habits of Highly Effective People" (1989) mentions the importance of empathy and information in communique. By speaking in terms that the listener can recognize and relate to, we are growing a bridge, facilitating communication and function an effect on.

Returning to our vicinity of hobby, how does this look at to hypnosis? Well, it's miles easy. Hypnotic hints are, in essence, communique system. But in evaluation to everyday communique, they're designed to speak right now to the subconscious.

It's as if you have been talking to a friend in a loud café. To get him to be aware of you, you want to beautify your voice, be easy and direct. Similarly, hypnotic hints are designed to "upward thrust above the noise," to pierce the conscious mind and communicate without delay to the unconscious. And to try this correctly, you need the right terms, the proper tone and, most significantly, the right context and intention.

But what precisely does it endorse to have the "proper aim"? In our next segment, we will delve greater deeply into this concern consider, exploring how terms, sponsored via the right aim, can grow to be tools for transformation. For now, I invite you to reflect on the electricity of your non-public terms and recollect how you operate them in your each day existence. For, due to the fact the logician Lao-Tse said inside the "Tao Te Ching" (sixth century B.C.), "Kind terms are clean to talk, but their echoes are infinitely lasting."

So, here we're, exploring the fascinating worldwide of language and its ability. Now, it is crucial to recognize the "purpose" in the back of the terms, due to the reality, as you will see, phrases on my own are not magic. It is the purpose behind them that makes them so effective. But first, allow's turn to a sensible instance to demonstrate this thing.

Imagine masters of hypnosis in a theater. They every say to a volunteer exactly the identical word: "When I depend range to three, you may sense a surge of happiness." However, one hypnotist says it with hesitation, at the same time as the alternative says it with deep self assurance and fact. The give up end result may be substantially one-of-a-type due to the intention in the lower back of their phrases.

Intentions are similar to the conductor inside the again of a symphony of terms. You could have the nice track, the quality musicians, however without a conductor who is aware of when and a way to conduct every section, the tune will not reap its entire ability.

Dr. Milton Erickson, taken into consideration by way of many to be the father of modern hypnosis and quoted in his famous paintings "My Voice Will Go With You" (1982), modified into a master within the use of motive. Not pleasant did he cautiously choose out his terms, however every word have become imbued with a purpose, a clean reason.

Now, allow's have a take a look at an instance of the manner motive combines with phrases to create an effective hypnotic notion.

Suppose you need to assist a person overcome their fear of public speaking. You might say, "Every time you stand in front of an purpose market, you experience assured and snug." Now, those phrases are critical, but with out a clean aim inside the returned of them, they simply flow in the air. In assessment, if you say that phrase with a deep perception and preference to make that individual actually experience assured and comfortable, the ones phrases deliver a totally unique weight. It is as in case you are sending the ones phrases immediately into the coronary coronary heart and thoughts of the listener.

Now, for the ones skeptics who may despite the fact that be questioning, "Is it really that clean?", it's far important to point out that simplicity is devious. As Albert Einstein said in a letter to Hans Muehsam in 1951, "Things need to be made as easy as possible, however now not easier." Hypnosis, with its wordplay and subtleties, is a smooth example of this.

So I invite you, high priced reader, to reflect onconsideration on your non-public life and how you talk your intentions through your words. Are you saying what you virtually recommend? Are you conveying your actual intentions? And most significantly, how need to you use the energy of goal to decorate your verbal exchange and persuasion competencies?

In our next segment, we are capable of delve even deeper into the artwork of blending phrases with intentions and the way those hints may be implemented in practical conditions. With examples, theory and a sprint of humor, we are able to dive into the charming international of language and its capability to transform our lives.

As we preserve our journey via the depths of language, we come across a few thing essential: the choice of our words. That's right, choice. It isn't enough to truely say a few thing; it must be said with precision, with aim and with reason. For on occasion, the slightest trade in phrase preference need to make a sizeable difference in its impact.

Think of it this way: there are more than 100 and seventy,000 phrases within the English dictionary, but the key is understanding which phrases to apply and even as to apply them. And once in a while it is not the phrase itself, but how it is said. It's that tone, that rhythm, that emphasis

reflect on the entirety we've were given explored. From the cause inside the returned of the words to the selection of terms, every piece of data has been designed to lead you to a deeper facts of the energy of language.

And in case you expect this adventure has been eye-starting up so far, I promise you that what is coming in the next financial ruin may be even greater eye-organising. We'll delve into rapid hypnosis techniques, those strategies that might positioned a person right into a trance state in minutes, every now and then even seconds. You will not satisfactory find out how they artwork, however additionally a way to exercising them in practical conditions. And with the useful resource of the use of reading the ones strategies, I promise you will have to your arms the tools to convert no longer best your every day interactions, however your existence as an entire.

So, are you ready to move forward and loose up even more secrets and techniques of the strength of hypnosis and language? I sit up straight for seeing you in the subsequent bankruptcy, in which discovery and transformation appearance ahead to you.

Chapter 5: Top five Most Effective Rapid Hypnosis Techniques

Imagine for a moment which you are shielding on your hands a container of magical gear. These are not any ordinary tools; they may be the grasp keys that could free up the doors of your thoughts, allowing you to get admission to power you failed to even apprehend you had. It's a charming concept, is not it? Well, the fact is which you do no longer need to imagine it. Because it's miles exactly what we're going to discover on this monetary destroy: the simplest and effective fast hypnosis strategies that could exchange your lifestyles in techniques you in no way imagined.

But why is it so crucial to understand those techniques? Let me pose you a query: Have you ever attempted to analyze a skills or damage a addiction and felt trapped, as even though there was an invisible wall preventing you from shifting ahead? Have you ever felt that there may be a higher version of yourself equipped to be released, however you sincerely cannot discover the vital component? Therein lies the power of rapid hypnosis. It is that key that unlocks your latent ability.

Hypnosis has been used for masses of years, from historic Egyptian cultures to modern treatment clinics. But in recent times, thanks to advances in neuroscience and statistics of the human mind, we've got subtle those strategies to be even extra powerful and effective.

Have you ever stopped to take into account the wonder that is your mind? It is more powerful than any supercomputer, greater mysterious than any unsolved enigma. It is a universe unto itself, full of goals, goals, fears and untapped ability. Carl Jung, in "Man and His Symbols" (1964), showed us how our psyche is product of layers and layers of content material material, a few conscious and a few now not. What if you could solve the ones mysteries, get to the ones deep layers and make enormous modifications in an immediate? The well data is that you could. And this financial ruin is your first step on that thrilling journey.

Before we dive into the strategies, allow me percentage a humorous anecdote that clarifies the concept. Two younger fish had been swimming after they handed an older fish coming inside the opposite path. The older fish said to them, "Hey guys, how's the water?". The young fish saved swimming for a while after which really one among them looked at the other and stated, "What the heck is water?" Sometimes the maximum apparent aspect is what escapes us the maximum!

Rapid hypnosis strategies, like water for fish, are ubiquitous factors that have constantly been there, waiting to be located and used for our benefit. They are mechanisms that, at the identical time as used well, can help you immerse your self in an altered u . S . A . Of cognizance, allowing you to get admission to that significant ocean of opportunities that is dwelling inner you.

So, are you equipped to dive into the depths of your mind and discover that strength inside you? Are you equipped to convert the version of your self you apprehend and take a quantum leap into an higher version? If your answer is wonderful, I encourage you to take a look at on and embark on one of the maximum captivating and transformative journeys of your existence. Because, ultimately, the energy has normally been on your arms; you clearly want the right equipment to unleash it.

Having set up the importance of what is at stake and the way effective those techniques may be, allow's delve into the fascinating global of fast hypnosis. Imagine having device to your repertoire that can reason change in a recollect of minutes. We're now not speaking about magic pointers, however real human thoughts magic.

Dr. Milton Erickson, one of the maximum renowned hypnotherapists of the 20th century, advocated a more naturalistic, solution-orientated hypnosis. In his e-book My Voice Will Accompany You (1982), Erickson stocks endless anecdotes approximately how he used diffused strategies to bring his sufferers into deep trance states. Erickson believed that each character has the solutions to their very very own problems; they actually need the right steerage to get proper of entry to them. And this is wherein rapid hypnosis strategies prove their actually well worth.

Magnetic Hand Induction: One of the most traditional strategies. Ask the situation to close their eyes and keep in mind that your palms are like effective magnets. As you talk and describe the magnetic attraction, the task will revel in your palms slowly begin to bypass nearer together. As the hands get closer, the thoughts dives deeper and deeper into the trance.

Staring Technique: Here an item is used, regularly a luminous issue or a pendulum. By asking the man or woman to maintain their gaze regular on that item, their attention narrows, allowing high-quality stimuli to vanish away. Essentially, you create a kingdom of hyperfocus that acts as a portal to trance.

If you have got got got ever observe "The Principles of Psychology" (1890) through the use of William James, you can encounter a quote that proclaims: "The best discovery of any generation is that someone can exchange his lifestyles via changing his thoughts-set". And that is precisely what fast hypnosis accomplishes. Through the ones techniques, an individual may be guided to adopt a present day day thoughts-set, a contemporary body of reference, in the blink of an eye fixed.

Let's hold with our listing.

3. Confusion Induction: This technique is based absolutely totally on momentarily difficult the conscious thoughts, which allows the subconscious thoughts to take over. By the usage of complicated language patterns or contradictory instructions, the aware thoughts is beaten, permitting the hypnotic u . S . To emerge.

four. Loss of Balance Induction: By slightly affecting the scenario's balance, it is possible to cause a rustic of vulnerability. The thoughts actually seeks a state of equilibrium and stability. By traumatic it bodily, an possibility is created to activate a trance.

It is captivating how the ones techniques, which can also additionally additionally seem clean or perhaps trivial within the starting look, have the power to get entry to the depths of the mind. It is a reminder of the truth that regularly the only solutions are not generally the maximum complicated.

5. The "Shock" Technique: By supplying the priority with a marvel or sudden stimulus, a short-time period void is created within the thoughts. This small vicinity, this pause, is the first-class opportunity to insert a hypnotic idea.

These strategies, while effective, are quality the stop of the iceberg. There are numerous different techniques, every tailored to wonderful individuals and situations. The critical difficulty is understanding and exercising.

The beauty of these strategies lies of their versatility and the way they may be incorporated into regular life. Imagine being able to calm your thoughts earlier than an important presentation, conquer a fear of flying in a don't forget of mins, or even improve your focus before a vital mission, for the duration of the use of speedy hypnosis.

Now in case you are wondering, "This sounds charming, but is it without a doubt for me?" allow me assure you that it is. Every individual has the ability to benefit from hypnosis. It's an innate functionality, some thing we've got all professional on some level, whether or not or now not or now not it is getting lost in a ebook, a film, or truely daydreaming.

So, are you prepared to delve similarly into this exciting worldwide? Because what comes subsequent will surprise you even more. And in case you enjoy this resonates with you, I promise the subsequent phase will take you even further for your journey to awakening your inner power.

The beauty of the human mind is its ability to comply and change. Our neuroplasticity, the thoughts's capability to reorganize itself and form new neural connections sooner or later of life, is really notable. But how can we harness this innate extremely good and combine it with speedy hypnosis strategies to collect even greater high-quality consequences?

The famous neuropsychologist Oliver Sacks, in his artwork "The Man Who Mistook His Wife for a Hat" (1985), provides a sequence of clinical times that display the brilliant resilience and adaptability of the human thoughts. Although Sacks did now not attention specifically on hypnosis, his observations at the thoughts's capacity to overcome disturbing conditions are profoundly relevant here.

Let's take a concrete example: that of an individual who suffers from immoderate anxiety in advance than public speaking. It's a situation that many face and it may be paralyzing. But what if we want to apply speedy hypnosis to reprogram that response?

Imagine, if you may, standing on a level. You feel the load of the target audience's stares on you. But in area of the acquainted worry, you experience a serene calm. Every time you breathe in, a experience of self guarantee fills you, and on every occasion you breathe out, you allow circulate of any trace of doubt. This is the electricity of rapid hypnosis in movement.

Dr. Richard Bandler, in his art work "The Structure of Magic" (1975), co-written with John Grinder, talks approximately the ability to change our emotional responses. Bandler indicates that if we're able to recognize the "shape" of the manner we create our internal realities, then we are able to alternate them.

Continuing with our instance, the character should use the Magnetic Hand Induction method to enter a country of rest. Once in that u . S ., he must visualize a a success beyond public speech, remembering each detail, each feeling. And then, he need to "switch" those powerful emotions to the modern-day situation, remodeling his reaction to the state of affairs.

In addition, the Staring technique should help the person attention on the winning second, getting rid of distractions and concerns about the judgment of others.

These aren't truly pretty theories. They are sensible techniques, sponsored through using manner of some years of research and exercise in the region of hypnotherapy.

The power of speedy hypnosis also can be visible in its capability to overcome trauma. As Bessel van der Kolk explains in "The Body Keeps Score" (2014), trauma can emerge as "trapped" inside the body, manifesting in physical and emotional symptoms. Rapid hypnosis offers a way to access and reprocess these stressful reminiscences.

Let's take any other instance, this time of a person who has had a demanding enjoy with water and has advanced a fear of water. Using Confusion Induction, we ought to take that individual to a country wherein the stressful reminiscences are tons much less "blanketed" with the resource of aware defenses. Once in that state, we need to guide her through a sequence of extraordinary visualizations, converting the disturbing recollections with new, extra empowering recollections.

Isn't it fascinating? The functionality is widespread. However, like numerous powerful device, it's miles essential to apply speedy hypnosis responsibly and continuously with the difficulty's well-being in mind.

Now, as you cross deeper into this financial destroy, I invite you to open your mind and your coronary coronary coronary heart to the opportunities. Every approach, every tale, each instance is an invite to find out the terrific capability of your very personal thoughts. And keep in mind, you are usually genuinely one concept some distance from transformational alternate.

As Milton H. Erickson, one of the maximum renowned figures in the worldwide of hypnotherapy, knew properly, the subconscious thoughts is a reservoir of statistics and abilities. In his influential artwork "Beyond Ericksonian Therapy" (1980), he compelled the significance of harnessing this subconscious power to promote profound and lasting adjustments in people. But what if I informed you that what we've got got explored thus far is best the pinnacle of the iceberg?

Let's have a look at it this way: If the mind have been an ocean, the quick hypnosis strategies we've got referred to will be the waves on the floor, seen and tangible. But there are deeper, greater mysterious and powerful currents geared up to be observed. The query is, are you ready to dive deeper?

As we've got were given navigated the strategies of speedy hypnosis, we've had been given mounted a strong basis. The waves, of route, have their power and beauty, however it's far within the depths in which the real treasure is located.

James Braid, considered by means of manner of the usage of many to be the "father of current-day hypnosis," positioned it elegantly in his paintings "Neurypnology" (1843), arguing that, thru hypnosis, one can also moreover want to get proper of get entry to to deeper layers of the mind, those darkish and frequently forgotten corners that disguise secrets and techniques and solutions.

So, having explored the floor, it is time for us to dive into the depths of self-hypnosis within the next chapter. Imagine, if you can, being in complete manipulate of your mind, being capable of get right of entry to those inner property each time you need to, and all this using the most effective device you personal: your very own thoughts.

What if I knowledgeable you that self-hypnosis permits you to be each the hypnotist and the undertaking, providing you with top notch autonomy to your method of self-exploration and transformation? Would you want to discover ways to harness that strength for yourself?

Before I finish this financial ruin, I want to depart you with a idea. Rapid hypnosis is truly a powerful and transformative approach, but remember that it is best one of many equipment for your arsenal. As with the entirety in life, practice and determination are key. The more you exercise and immerse yourself on this information, the deeper your understanding is probably and the more first-rate the adjustments you will experience.

So, high priced reader, are you ready to embark on this adventure of self-empowerment and discovery? In the subsequent financial ruin, we are capable of open the door to self-hypnosis, a talent that, as speedy as mastered, has the capability to transform your lifestyles in tactics you may every so often keep in thoughts now.

I invite you to preserve this journey, to dive deeper, to find out and unleash the strength internal you. The subsequent financial disaster is actually throughout the corner, prepared with ensures of self-information and transformation. Do you dare to take the bounce?

Chapter 6: Self-Hypnosis

Have you ever perplexed why fine human beings appear to have extraordinary manage over their lives? Why, irrespective of what takes place, they appear to transport with grace, self warranty and resolution? I'll provide you with a touch: it's far now not magic, it's not achievement, and it's far genuinely now not due to the truth they're genetically talented. It's due to the reality they've got located and mastered a effective device, a device that everybody, which includes you, has inner of them Ready to discover?

Introducing self-hypnosis.

Self-hypnosis, because the call implies, is hypnosis directed at you. It is the planned act of having access to your subconscious and making changes to your concept patterns, conduct and ideals. Imagine being on pinnacle of things of an internal operating gadget, tailoring it to behave constant together with your desires and goals. Fascinating, isn't always it?

But why is this tool so important? Well, for the duration of your existence, you have got got obtained beliefs, attitudes and behaviors primarily based in your stories, schooling and way of life. Some of these styles are useful and serve you nicely. Others, however, restrict you. You might not also be privy to them, however they may be there, performing as an invisible script that directs your conduct.

Now, remember being capable of rewrite that script, replace it and optimize it to better reflect who you're and in that you need to head. Self-hypnosis gives you that ability. It is, in essence, a form of self-development this is going past easy motivation. It is ready reprogramming your mind.

You may think, "Ah! But I've already tried to change and function not succeeded." I apprehend. However, let me ask you some factor: Have you attempted to do it from the internal out? Because it certainly is the splendor of self-hypnosis. It's not handiest a relaxation or meditation method. It's a way for alternate from the premise.

Of direction, you do now not just have to take my word for it. In "The Power of Now" (1997), Eckhart Tolle talks approximately the power of the winning and the significance of spotting and changing our intellectual styles. Although his approach is typically spiritual, there may be a deep connection to the act of self-hypnosis: being privy to your mind and taking active manage over them.

If you are questioning approximately the relevance of self-hypnosis in the modern-day worldwide, keep in thoughts this: We live in an age of consistent distractions.

Social media, news, work, own family... All compete for our interest. Self-hypnosis, then, isn't first-class a tool for converting antique patterns, however additionally a way for finding clarity and focus in a chaotic global.

Remember while we said recommendations in Chapter 4? Well, with self-hypnosis, you could supply recommendations to your self. Imagine the opportunities. And sure, in case you suppose this sounds too first rate to be actual, it certainly is understandable. But I task you to embark on this journey, to discover for your self the transformative electricity of self-hypnosis. After all, what do you have to lose and what sort of do you stand to benefit?

To close to this advent, I depart you with a chunk of light humor: Why hypnotists are so appropriate at activities? Because they normally comprehend the manner to set off the "birthday party mode" in human beings's minds! And with self-hypnosis, you could additionally learn how to prompt any "mode" you need on your private mind.

So, as we preserve to unravel the wonders of self-hypnosis, I need you to consider a few factor. If you have been in popular manage of your mind, what's going to be the number one trouble you may trade? Think difficult, because of the truth that concept may be the start of your transformation. And in the next segment, we are capable of go even deeper into the brilliant worldwide of self-hypnosis. I promise you it is going to be a fascinating adventure.

If you have got ever confused how lots control you certainly have over your thoughts, this is the time at the same time as we're going to dig even deeper. The human thoughts is a complex surprise, and what is at stake is its nearly limitless capability for change and model. Once you apprehend this energy, you'll apprehend that you'll be the hold close of your personal destiny.

Throughout facts, awesome thinkers and leaders have understood the significance of understanding and controlling the mind. Napoleon Hill in "Think and Grow Rich" (1937) writes approximately the have an impact on of our thoughts on our movements and the way they without delay have an impact on our results. This is a lesson that resonates even more when we communicate about self-hypnosis. If you can trade your mind, you may trade your moves, and therefore, your life.

This is wherein self-hypnosis becomes a beneficial device. But how exactly does it paintings? Well, maintain in mind your thoughts as an iceberg. The detail you spot above the surface of the water is your conscious thoughts. This is the detail you use to make each day choices, have a examine statistics and reason. However, the large mass that lies underneath the water, hidden from view, is your unconscious mind. This is in which your ingrained beliefs, reminiscences and feelings are placed. And accept as authentic with it or no longer, it's far this underwater issue that during big part drives your each day conduct.

Self-hypnosis, then, is the technique of speaking right away with that submerged detail. It is a way to dive deep, enter into communicate collectively along with your unconscious and make modifications at a vital level. And certain, this may sound a piece mystical, however it's miles a exercising sponsored by way of manner of era.

Dr. James Braid, taken into consideration through many to be the daddy of modern-day-day hypnosis, have become one of the first to apprehend the significance of this altered state of consciousness. In his paintings "Neurypnology" (1843), Braid describes how hypnosis can be used to get admission to forgotten memories, trade behaviors, and normally have an impact on the human thoughts in previously no longer feasible techniques.

So, if you're sitting there, wondering, "This all sounds high-quality, however how do I are aware about it is actual?". I pay hobby you. It's natural to be skeptical, specifically close to a few element as precis and esoteric because the human mind. But generation is on our side.

For example, more than one research have established that self-hypnosis may be powerful in hundreds of packages, from pain remedy to improving athletic basic overall performance. Functional magnetic resonance imaging techniques, which map thoughts interest, show actual modifications inside the mind in a few unspecified time within the future of hypnotic states. This isn't magic or pseudoscience. It is the real and tested power of the human mind in movement.

And a hint comic interlude to lighten the mood: What's the maximum exciting interest within the worldwide? Hypnotist! After all, they're continually putting humans to sleep!

Getting again to the main topic, I want you to think about some thing. We all have behaviors or conduct that we would love to change. Maybe it is an addiction to candies, procrastination or everyday self-doubt. What if I informed you that, with self-hypnosis, you could start to cope with and change the ones behaviors at their root?

Of direction, it is not a miracle remedy. You won't emerge as a contemporary day individual in a single day. But with workout and staying power, self-hypnosis may be that tool that takes you to the following diploma on your journey of self-discovery and boom.

In the subsequent phase, we're able to explore how you can start running toward self-hypnosis and a few practical examples a terrific manner to visualise its software program in actual lifestyles. Because, at the give up of the day, it is not quite an lousy lot principle and philosophy. It's about movement. It's about trade. And you have were given the power to make it take location.

Let's speak about how, precisely, you can begin to exercise self-hypnosis. By immersing ourselves within the ones tactics, we're seeking out a way to installation a right away line of conversation with that big and powerful unconscious we had been talking about. It is time to prevent being spectators and become administrators of our non-public highbrow film.

Imagine for a second that you are within the the front of a large mansion. This mansion represents your mind. Have you visited all the rooms? Do all its secrets and techniques and techniques and strategies? Do you recognize what's hidden in its darkest corners? With self-hypnosis, you will become the explorer of this majestic palace, coming across its wonders and going via its mysteries.

And here, I will provide you with a maintain close key. But, in advance than you challenge into the mansion, it's far crucial to recognize positive thoughts.

In his e-book "The Power of Your Subconscious Mind" (1963), Joseph

Murphy delves into how the unconscious absorbs statistics and the way, via repetition and popularity, we can have an impact on it. This precept is the middle of self-hypnosis. It is ready repetition, recognition and, especially, intention.

1. Choose your goal: Whether you need to get rid of a terrible habit, enhance your self belief or certainly loosen up, you have to have a clean purpose in mind in advance than you begin.

2. Find a quiet region: A quiet environment with out distractions is important. The proper surroundings makes it less difficult to get right of entry in your unconscious.

three. Deep relaxation: Close your eyes, take a deep breath and visualize a staircase. With each step down, you enjoy an increasing number of snug, leaving within the decrease back of the tensions of regular life.

four. Induction: Use brilliant affirmations associated with your cause. Repeat them to your mind, with conviction and feeling.

five. Visualization: Imagine that you have already reached your aim. Feel the excitement, have a take a look at the facts. In this country, your unconscious mind does now not distinguish among fact and creativeness, so it absorbs this new "reality" you're growing.

6. Awakening: Count slowly from 1 to 5, telling your self that you will sense refreshed and renewed while you open your eyes.

Now, a concrete instance. Suppose you want to overcome your fear of public speaking. After exciting, visualize yourself inside the front of an audience, feeling consistent, assured. Listen to the applause, watch the smiles of approval. Each time you workout this visualization, you will be reinforcing for your unconscious the concept which you are a equipped and confident speaker.

Remember whilst we noted in Chapter 4 about the energy of words? Well, this is wherein that information plays a important position. Your affirmations and visualizations inside the path of self-hypnosis must be smooth and effective, averting any terrible language.

And, if you're wondering in case you've ever been under self-hypnosis without figuring out it, the solution is a effective "sure." Have you ever been so immersed in a e-book or film that the outside global appears to vanish away? That's a form of hypnotic trance. The distinction now is which you have the equipment to go into that America of the usa at will and direct it towards your dreams.

Let us skip on. In the subsequent segment, we're able to delve greater deeply into the results and possibilities of self-hypnosis. Because when you maintain near this ability, the opportunities are certainly countless. And it is also thrilling to count on, "What else can I accomplish?" Let's find out together!

Chapter 7: Tactics against Stress and Anxiety

Have you ever felt like a stress cooker, equipped to blow up at the slightest stimulus? Or perhaps you have felt like a butterfly trapped in a spider's net, not capable of transport below the weight of stress and anxiety? If you're nodding your head, you are now not by myself. These feelings, whilst natural, may be hard if now not managed nicely but what if I knowledgeable you that there are strategies to launch that strain and manipulate anxiety in mins? What if you can do it without medicine, years of remedy and without spending a fortune?

In the twenty first century, the urgency of modern-day life, era and the normal call for to be "connected" have exacerbated the ones feelings. Selye (1974) in "The Stress of Life" tells us that strain is the "seasoning of life," however what happens at the same time as that seasoning turns into the number one path? Remember in Chapter 4 while we noted the strength of phrases? Here, too, they play a vital role. The manner we talk and bear in mind ourselves can be the distinction amongst dwelling under a black cloud of pressure or on foot round with the solar shining on our heads.

Mental unblocking is not honestly a method; it's miles a manner of lifestyles. It is the recognition that our thoughts has the capacity to manipulate and redecorate our emotions and reactions, in area of being slaves to them.

For a second, I need you to consider a time while you felt quite stressed or aggravating. Do you have got that image to your thoughts? Now, I need you to hold in thoughts what befell honestly earlier than that 2nd. Was it a communication, a perception, an picture, or a experience?

These are called "triggers" and are vital to information a manner to approach intellectual unblocking.

Now, replicate for a 2d: what if we want to learn how to recognize and reply to the ones triggers in advance than they grow to be an avalanche of emotions? That is exactly what you can look at in this bankruptcy.

Did you already know that in 1962, Victor Frankl, in his art work "Man's Search for Meaning", stated that among stimulus and reaction there can be a space? And in that area lies our freedom and potential to select out our reaction. Rapid hypnosis offers us with the device to amplify that place, giving us greater time and clarity to select how we need to answer.

Before I continue, I want you to mirror on some thing: how usually an afternoon do you are taking a second to pause and really breathe? If your answer is "now not many," you aren't on my own. Most humans circulate thru life on autopilot, reacting in vicinity of responding. But proper here's the good data: with the strategies you'll studies on this financial disaster, you may not handiest be capable of unblock your thoughts in mins, but you can moreover emerge as the draw close of your emotions.

As we dive deeper into this bankruptcy, we're going to find out unique techniques that will help you understand and neutralize those triggers, offering you with a experience of manage and freedom. Are you geared up to interrupt loose from the chains of pressure and anxiety? Because you're about to embark on one of the maximum interesting journeys of your existence.

If you're curious about what is coming next, it's far a sign which you're equipped for exchange. And, if you're thinking how all this compares to what we've got got already stated approximately self-hypnosis in Chapter 6, absolutely wait until you be aware how those strategies interconnect and make bigger the benefits. Let's dive deeper into the first rate international of highbrow unblocking!

And, as I predicted, intellectual unblocking is a great deal greater than a simple trick. It is an entire renewal of wondering, a reconfiguration of the thoughts. Think of it as a spring cleansing to your thoughts.

Have you ever found how our minds often experience like a dusty attic full of vintage containers of memories, some of which we don't even keep in mind we had? Well, pressure and tension techniques are equipment to help you dust, reorganize and, most importantly, put off what now not serves you.

Now, Richard Bandler and John Grinder in "The Structure of Magic" (1975) provide an reason behind how terms create truth. If we continuously tell ourselves that we're confused or traumatic, what do you located will seem? It will become our fact. But what if we should exchange that internal speech?

Imagine that every bad belief is kind of a crumpled sheet of paper. If you maintain crumpling the sheet over and over, it turns into a compact, unwieldy ball. But in case you take a moment to smooth it out, to undo those wrinkles, the sheet becomes possible all over again. That's how highbrow unblocking works: it smoothes out those wrinkled mind, making them less complex to deal with.

One of the primary steps to intellectual unblocking is mastering to end up aware of the ones horrible thoughts. Did that, consistent with Aaron T. Beck in "Cognitive

Therapy and Emotional Disorders" (1976), most people have among 12,000 and 60,000 mind a day, and 80% of those are terrible? That's an amazing quantity of negativity! But worry no longer, because of the reality with the proper techniques; you may flip those thoughts in your benefit.

Start through the usage of journaling your mind. Yes, I understand what you are wondering, "Another magazine?" But accept as authentic with me, this one can be one in every of a kind. It's now not about writing down what you possibly did during the day, but the way you felt and what mind you had. Once you begin identifying the ones terrible thoughts, you could paintings on changing them.

Now, undergo in mind in Chapter 5 whilst we pointed out fast hypnosis techniques. Well, this is in which they come into play. Using those strategies, you could reprogram the ones horrible thoughts, turning them into superb affirmations. For example, in place of telling yourself "I cannot do that," strive "I truly have all the equipment I want to satisfy this mission." See the difference.

And, of path, respiratory performs a critical position in all of this. Remember once I referred to taking pauses to breathe? Well, at the identical time as you feel pressure and tension taking on, take a 2nd to shut your eyes, take a deep breath and repeat your quality affirmations. It's wonderful how powerful it is able to be.

Do you laugh at the idea? I apprehend it sounds clean, and in many techniques it is. But as Leonardo da Vinci stated, "simplicity is the very last sophistication." Sometimes, the best solutions are the great. And in our quest to free up the thoughts, every so often all we need is to consider to breathe.

It's an exquisite feeling to apprehend which you have the electricity to alternate your truth surely through manner of changing your thoughts. And while it is able to no longer take place in a unmarried day, with exercise and backbone, I guarantee you will see results. So, are you organized to dive even deeper into those techniques? Because there may be so much extra to find out.

Understanding and coping with emotions is vital to any highbrow unblocking approach. Consider your feelings as symptoms on a control board. If a trademark lights up, you don't forget approximately it; you determine out what is going on. Emotions are the ones symptoms, and know-how them is fundamental to having a clean and loose mind.

But it is not just about expertise your private feelings. It is essential to discover ways to empathize and understand the emotions of others, as this may immediately have an impact on your intellectual nicely-being. Daniel Goleman in "Emotional Intelligence" (1995) argued that the ability to recognize, understand and manage our feelings, and moreover understand and understand the emotions of others, is crucial to our ordinary achievement in life. The perfect information is that, like many special skills, this can be placed out and improved with exercise.

Let me allow you to recognize a tale. Samuel have become a person who modified into regularly beaten through his emotions. Stressful conditions at paintings, arguments collectively along along with his accomplice, and financial problems regularly made him revel in like he turned into in a pressure cooker. These situations introduced about excessive emotional responses in him, which then affected his potential to suppose in truth and make rational alternatives.

Samuel determined to are on the lookout for for assist and started out to have a take a look at particular meditation and self-hypnosis strategies. One day, at the same time as education a respiration method, he had a second of revelation. He located out that it changed into not the conditions themselves which have been inflicting his pressure and anxiety, but his reaction to the ones conditions.

From then on, whenever he determined himself in a stressful scenario, Samuel should save you for a 2d, take a deep breath and visualize a wave in the ocean. He imagined that his emotions have been that wave, powerful and overwhelming before the entirety, but ultimately fading into the shore, leaving calm inside the back of. This visualization helped her to unblock her mind and technique conditions with a clearer and calmer attitude.

Can you grow to be privy to with Samuel? Many people undergo similar situations, and the key is to discover ways to respond, not react. When you reply, you're making a aware choice approximately how to act, while reacting is an automatic impulse. And as we said in Chapter four, the power of terms and the manner we communicate to ourselves can also have a profound effect on our mind-set.

In addition, visualization carrying activities may be distinctly effective for highbrow unblocking. For example, keep in mind a non violent river. Each concept or fear is a leaf floating down that river. Instead of trying to capture and study every leaf, in truth watch them glide away, leaving you in a kingdom of peace and clarity.

While those strategies can also sound too smooth, do no longer underestimate their energy. As Eckhart Tolle would possibly say in "The Power of Now" (1997), the winning 2nd is all we truly have, and getting to know to be actually present can be a effective device for highbrow unblocking.

So, are you inclined to make the leap and discover ways to manage your emotions in preference to permitting them to manipulate you? Because while you do, you will discover a whole new worldwide of possibilities.

Having already explored the sizeable universe of emotions, intellectual blocks and strategies for coping with them, it is time to dive a bit deeper into how all of these interrelate within the difficult net of our thoughts. Carl Gustav Jung as soon as said, in his art work "Psychological Types" (1921), that "until you are making the aware subconscious, it'll direct your life and you can call it destiny." This word consists of with it a weight that can be deeply felt in facts the connection amongst our aware and subconscious mind.

As we navigate thru the meanderings of the human mind, permit's preserve in mind how Samuel used visualization to calm his inner hurricane. Now, do not forget being capable of do that, however at an wonderful deeper stage. Consider the vast strength you could have if you could channel your energies and manage your responses, now not clearly in stressful conditions, but in all factors of your existence. What if I knowledgeable you that the following step for your adventure ought to lead you to exactly that capability?

There's a worldwide indoors you ready to be discovered, a gold mine of untapped functionality. But, like each mine, it is able to be tricky to navigate with out the proper system. So what device is more effective than controlling and data your non-public goals?

Think about your desires for a 2nd. Have you ever woken up from a dream and felt that it had an crucial message for you, however you had been no longer certain what it changed into? Dreams are the gateway to the subconscious, and analyzing to interpret and paintings with them can be the vital thing to unlocking potentials you did not even understand you had.

You've already come an prolonged manner, but the adventure is without a doubt beginning. In the next monetary smash, we are capable of delve into the captivating global of "Hypnosis and Sleep," in which you may discover ways to reprogram your thoughts at the same time as you sleep, tapping into the thoughts's awesome functionality to heal, look at and grow within the realm of desires. By studying those techniques, you may recognise that the sky is not the restrict; in reality, your mind is the restriction.

So I ask you: are you equipped to evoke in a worldwide in which every night time gives you the possibility to increase and remodel? I guarantee you that when you discover the secrets and techniques behind the veil of sleep, you may in no manner take a look at bedtime the identical way again. I stay up for seeing you within the next financial disaster, wherein the celebrities of your desires will moderate up the route for your real self.

Chapter 8: Reprogramming Your Nocturnal Subconscious

You've tasted the sweet nectar of rest after a protracted day, proper? But have you ever ever ever stopped to take into account the amazing theater that unfolds in your thoughts every night time time time time on the identical time as you sleep? And no, I'm not actually speakme approximately those fanciful goals in which you fly over surreal landscapes or become the protagonist of an motion film. I'm talking about the massive unconscious world ready to be determined, explored and, most importantly, tapped into.

Why, you ask, want to I care what is going on in my mind when I am napping? Let me answer your question with every different question: If you had an incredibly effective gadget, may additionally need to you leave it unattended all night time, every night time? Of direction you would no longer. So why can we permit our minds, one of the most effective machines recognized to mankind, to run without actual purpose throughout one of the most vital durations of recovery and rejuvenation?

Since time immemorial, philosophers, scientists and thinkers have been interested in dreams. Sigmund Freud, in "The Interpretation of Dreams" (1900), postulated that dreams are a manifestation of our unconscious dreams, a replicate reflecting the darkest and most hidden recesses of our psyche. But beyond symbolic interpretations, there can be a practical functionality inside the dream that loads of us have not considered.

And the fact is that, every night time, whilst we sleep, our mind does no longer near down, but shifts gears. It engages in a way of consolidation, processing and, what is maximum applicable to us on this bankruptcy, programming. Imagine, for a second, that each night time you have got got the possibility to reconfigure and application your unconscious mind. What could you change? What should you enhance? What new capabilities or perspectives should you want to domesticate?

Throughout this bankruptcy, we are capable of find out the massive energy behind the connection among hypnosis and sleep. If in preceding chapters you determined a manner to unblock your mind and combat pressure (check out Chapter 7 if you need a refresher), you are now approximately to embark on a adventure at the way to will assist you to do simply that, but on the private and most private diploma feasible.

Sleep isn't always pleasant a passive period of inactiveness. It is a doorway, a gateway to a worldwide wherein some thing is possible. What if I informed you that you may learn how to be the director of your private midnight movie, that you may script and orchestrate your desires to paintings on your determine on? No, this is not technological know-how fiction or fable. It is a systematic fact and a device that, with the right steering, is at your fingertips.

So, luxurious reader, are you organized to end up the architect of your desires? Are you geared up to harness the electricity of the night time time and shape your destiny at the same time as you sleep? Think approximately it. Night is proper right here, and with it, a golden possibility to reprogram your nocturnal unconscious. Darkness isn't always a void; it is a canvas, and you are approximately to turn out to be the artist.

As you maintain studying, you will find that the phrases go along with the drift with out troubles, that every idea connects to the subsequent, like portions of a splendidly designed puzzle. Relax, take a deep breath and put together to immerse your self inside the captivating global of hypnosis and dreaming. Because this night, you could not high-quality dream; you may redesign.

The dating among sleep and the unconscious is a mystery that has intrigued mankind considering the fact that time immemorial. When one plunges into the depths of sleep, the conscious relinquishes manipulate and allows the unconscious to take over. It is a international governed with the aid of way of felony pointers of its private, wherein the non-public desires, fears and aspirations come to lifestyles. A location that has end up the cornerstone of the maximum advanced research in hypnosis.

Dr. Michael Walker, in his e-book "The Internal Clock: Synchronizing Sleep with the Subconscious" (2012), describes how the mind operates in cycles at some level inside the night time time, transitioning amongst precise tiers of sleep. Each segment, Walker elements out, has a specific cause, from consolidation of recollections to mobile restore. But what truly captures our hobby is the REM section, that magical time on the same time as desires come to be greater brilliant and mind interest resembles that of a waking nation.

Have you ever notion approximately the endless possibilities this u . S . Offers, the ability to teach your mind to artwork on your behalf, make adjustments, red meat up amazing beliefs or maybe do away with blockages while you're in deep sleep?

The thoughts is plastic, malleable. Robert Winston, in "The Evolving Mind: The Power to Change" (2003), proposes that, with the proper stimulation, we will alternate the shape and feature of our neural networks. Now, reflect onconsideration on the REM segment as that maximum satisfying time to persuade this neuroplasticity. Hypnosis, with its capability to get entry to the subconscious, acts as the precise tool to orchestrate those modifications for the duration of sleep.

Imagine if you could take gain of that middle of the night window, that section at the same time as the thoughts is receptive and open, to enforce high-quality pointers. Do you want to enhance your vanity, possibly collect a modern talent or conquer an ingrained fear? The combination of hypnosis and sleep may be your passport to the ones achievements.

Of path, it is not only a do not forget of wishing for it. You want to use a way, a manner. Throughout this bankruptcy, we are able to introduce you to the techniques that the exceptional hypnotherapists within the worldwide have perfected to achieve this. And yes, you're in all likelihood feeling a piece skeptical. "How can that be?" you can ask. But, as Carl Sagan talked about in "The World and Its Demons" (1995), "Absence of evidence is not proof of absence." And whilst this vicinity continues to be below studies, the testimonials and fulfillment reminiscences speak for themselves.

The key's training and recognition. Before going to sleep, it's far important to create a conducive environment, away from distractions and charged with purpose. Don't neglect about, as we noted in Chapter 4, the power of phrases and the way they may act because of the truth the reason that devices off a series of automatic responses for your mind.

So how approximately beginning a brand new ritual this night time, a ritual that no longer great gives you a restful sleep, however moreover a transformative sleep? Because, at the forestall of the day, sleep isn't always only a rest; it is an opportunity, a door to a global of countless possibilities. And you, steeply-priced reader, preserve the essential aspect.

Continuing this journey through the mysteries of sleep and the unconscious, it is time to dive into concrete examples of the way hypnosis has stimulated this herbal country, leading to excellent effects.

Do you bear in mind ever waking up from a dream feeling that there was some thing in it which you had to bear in mind? As in case your thoughts emerge as presenting you with a clue, but it all seemed so remote and airy that you could not draw near its essence. Well, you aren't on my own in that enjoy. Sarah Thompson, a 28-

twelve months-antique female, positioned herself in a similar state of affairs. For years, she had time and again dreamed of a model of herself who performed the violin masterfully. Every time she wakened, she felt a deep connection to that instrument, notwithstanding the reality that she had in no way completed it in her lifestyles.

After analyzing approximately the functionality of hypnosis to enhance abilities and enhance mastering (a topic we are able to talk in addition in Chapter eleven), Sarah decided to attempt it for herself. She went to a hypnosis professional and, after numerous intervals geared toward reinforcing that connection the various dream and the choice to learn how to play the violin, she began her workout in the actual international.

The result became extraordinary. Not satisfactory did she have a study with astonishing pace, however she moreover felt that each time she picked up the violin, a surge of emotions and recollections from her goals flooded in, empowering her capacity. Sarah no longer exceptional wakened a today's passion but demonstrated the actual strength of sleep mixed with hypnosis.

This isn't always an isolated case. In his ebook "Lucid Dreaming and the Power of the Subconscious" (1998), Anthony Ross mentions numerous examples of folks that, with the useful aid of combining hypnosis strategies with lucid dreaming practices, were able to get right of entry to hidden potentials and clear up deep-seated private problems.

Of direction, consequences also can variety. As Ross says, "Not all goals are destined to emerge as display up realities, but every dream includes a seed of opportunity." And therein lies the magic. It is that seed that may be cultivated and nurtured thru hypnosis techniques, remodeling our dreamscape right proper right into a fertile garden for non-public growth.

Now, consider this. You are popularity in a massive library. Each ebook represents a night time's dream. By beginning considered one in each of them, you can assessment, examine and studies from the desires recorded in its pages. With the proper steerage, you could take that understanding and apply it to gain you in real lifestyles. Think about it for a moment: How tons of that ability, that full-size ocean of understanding and possibility, have you ever ever left unexplored?

If the idea is thrilling to you, you aren't by myself. Dr. Frederick Myles, in "Dream Connections: The Boundary Between Dream and Reality" (2015), highlights how cutting-edge-day studies is sincerely scratching the floor of what might be the next tremendous revolution in health and private development. By using hypnosis to get right of entry to that dream realm, we're able to begin to decipher the mysteries our thoughts gives us with night time after night time.

So, the following time you wake up from a dream, instead of simply forgetting approximately it and going on together along with your day, pause. Reflect. Ask your self, "What is my mind trying to tell me?" And in case you experience there can be a message or an functionality prepared to be located, maintain in mind which you have the system and the know-how to make it display up. Because, ultimately, each night time time you're immersed in a international of infinite opportunities. Isn't it time you began tapping into them?

With the diploma set, it is time to dive even deeper into the synergy among hypnosis and the sector of sleep. As in case you were floating on an ocean of possibilities, wherein every wave takes you to understand a deeper issue of your being, I invite you to discover this fascinating phenomenon with me.

Professor Leonard Hartsfield, in his have a take a look at "Intersections of Sleep and Hypnosis" (2002), said that "our mind is like an infinite e-book, where each internet web page contains tales and schooling we have however to discover." Through hypnosis, we've got the potential to have a study the ones pages consciously and intentionally, permitting desires, frequently mysterious and elusive, to become smooth and revealing.

So why is this hyperlink between sleep and hypnosis so essential? Imagine for a 2d that you have get proper of entry to to an infinite aid of data and self-expertise, but maximum of the time it is hidden within the lower back of a locked door. Hypnosis is that master key which can unfastened up that door, allowing you to get entry to the solutions and solutions that your subconscious has stored.

The stand-up comic and author, Mark Twain, as soon as quipped, "I've had pretty some issues in my life, most of which in no way befell." With this, he modified into highlighting how our minds regularly create situations primarily based completely mostly on fears and issues that never materialize. But what if you could face the ones scenarios inside the realm of your goals, prepare for them, and in the end triumph over them? It's an thrilling proposition, do not you suspect?

In addition to overcoming fears, the combination of hypnosis and sleep also can be a treasured tool for those looking for to beautify their abilties or analyze new ones. Imagine being capable of exercise a language, rehearse a speech or enlarge a knowledge while you sleep. The truth is that, with the right method and unique guidance, that is greater than feasible.

But I desire you won't in reality take my phrase for it. Dr. Miranda Greene, in "The Sleeping Consciousness: Discovering Dream Potential" (2017), describes in detail how the aware act of programming and guiding our goals can bring about no longer feasible personal and professional boom.

As you reflect on all that we've protected in this chapter, I choice you experience a spark of excitement and hobby, a choice to discover this effective and transformative device. Because, at the prevent of the day, the strength is residing within you, waiting to be unlocked.

And now, as you put together to embark on the subsequent financial ruin of this journey, I want to provide you a bit preview. In the following financial damage, we're going to address "The Mind-Body Link: Accelerated Healing and Vitality". Get prepared to discover how hypnosis can't nice have an effect to your thoughts, however additionally your frame, taking you to levels of health and health you can in no manner have imagined possible Ready for the following step on this transformative adventure? I promise, you may now not need to miss it.

Chapter 9: What about the Dangers of Hypnosis?

One of the reasons you pay interest about hypnosis is that, even for people who are untrained in the psycho dynamics of human conduct, it may be unstable.

Since best medical psychologists and psychiatrists have acquired great training in studying human conduct, this objection, if it's miles right, can also restrict hypnosis to a small enterprise organization of therapists who're comparably professional.

Thankfully, it is not actual this became validated a few years in the past while the Bride Murphy" craze took the kingdom by using storm. Little to no harm went into its killing in spite of the reality that loads of beginner hypnotists were the use of hypnosis.

I in truth have in my view professional plenty of scientific and non-scientific human beings, and I clearly have no longer but heard of a unmarried instance in which hypnosis led to a volatile or detrimental occasion that caused a catastrophe. I've also taught self hypnosis to hundreds of humans, and they might share the equal results.

Many sufferers who get preserve of professional treatment from psychologists, psychiatrists, and psychoanalysts won't continuously see high great outcomes. This does now not propose that human beings have to give up contacting those specialists for assistance. Not even a expert has a great music file of effective treatment.

But what precisely is the problem with hypnosis? The concept that removing one symptom will cause the emergence of a few other is commonly promoted with the useful resource of using humans with constrained or no historical past in hypnosis.

Differences of opinion do, however, exist even amongst folks who exercising hypnosis in this area. While a few hypnotists in reality do away with the symptom, others "change down" signs and symptoms thru substituting a intense symptom with a minor one.

When a health practitioner prescribes aspirin for arthritis, he does the latter. Although he's aware that aspirin won't cope with his arthritis, he nonetheless desires to control the symptom.

It is unscientific and pretend to claim that the pain will be replaced via manner of every other symptom.

Another grievance of hypnosis is that its results are best non permanent and symptomatic. It's vital to hold in mind that almost all of scientific treatment is meant to cast off signs and symptoms and symptoms.

What is the maximum everlasting clinical treatment? When you integrate self-hypnosis with hetero-hypnosis, you deliver the patient the chance to use the suggestions each time they will be desired for his very own gain.

Naturally, this could bring about prolonged-lasting symptom comfort. For instance, I do no longer see any harm in education a affected man or woman the way to hypnotize themselves in case you need to deal with their insomnia symptoms.

It might truely be most superb to physical depress the higher thoughts facilities with napping capsules each night time on the way to bring about unconsciousness.

You do not need me to tell you that tens of hundreds of thousands of dollars are spent yearly on sleeping remedy and that sufferers broaden dependent on them and require increasingly more pills to doze off. An overdose of dozing pills is the cause of many accidental suicides.

Nevertheless, loads of thousands of humans get prescriptions for snoozing tablets regardless of the obvious risks related to them, not to say individuals who get into the marketplace illegally.

Moreover, what is the real effort located forth to wean the affected man or woman off the drowsing capsules? Moreover, slumbering drugs are utilized in extra voluntary suicides than a few exceptional method.

If those drug treatments weren't so widely handy, possibly quite a few the ones unfortunate humans ought to nonetheless be with us nowadays.

What approximately the statement that is often quoted, particularly " consumer's personal moves can also additionally do some harm"?

Explore this place, please. I’m assuming that someone is aware of Emile Coupe’s art work to a degree or has heard of his well-known autosuggestion technique, which goes, Day thru day, in every way, I'm getting better and better.

Reciting this confirmation multiple times each day due to the truth the man or woman is going to sleep has helped plenty upon hundreds of instances in our time that regarded hopeless and helpless.

Regardless of the terminology used to explain it autosuggestion, excellent wondering, yoga, meditation, affirmations, or self-hypnosis I consider it is important to understand that we are all relating to the identical exercise. Before they're able to all function well for the man or woman, they all want to fulfill some critical necessities. These necessities can be blanketed in the upcoming bankruptcy.

It's essential to maintain in thoughts that the hints are stepping into the unconscious, which does now not test, doubt, examine, or contest the validity of those useful thoughts.

You may be sure that the continued exercise will undergo fruit. Hasn't society within the past identified everybody's

diagnosis on the time of "I'm ill, In How to Attain Self Hypnosis vein ferocity complex,

Is Ho How to Attain Self-Hypnosis A Ho How to Attain Self Hypnosis Attain Self Hypnosis t How to Attain Self-Hypnosis t How to Attain Self-Hypnosis cause Self-

Hypnosis ant prevent smoking," "Inca How to Attain Self-Hypnosis

Hypnosis o Hypnosis se weight, I find out it tough to go to sleep," "I absolutely cannot appear to loosen up,"

Isn't this individual successfully the usage of self, hasn't the character persuaded himself that his modern-day state of affairs is legitimate? This is extremely volatile. It is opposite hypnosis.

Whyshouldn'tthesubconsciousmindbeevenmoreconvincedandrespondstronglytosuggestionswhichareinconformitywiththenatural preference to be of sound frame and mind?" I've in no way been able to offer you with a practical response.

I accept as actual with that that is a commonplace incidence. A character is going to hypnosis for help with a problem that is clearly unrelated to hypnosis. His healing isn't reliant on being placed underneath hypnosis or on recommendations that he or the hypnotist deem crucial.

Every ebook and article approximately hypnosis that you take a look at will train you that hypnotism isn't a treatment all."

Nobody has made any indicators guidelines that it ought to be the most effective remedy used for emotional issues.

A newspaper article concerning the dangers of hypnosis can also have caught your interest.

It can also want to describe a person who professional one symptom after which developed every different instead.

Typically, you're given a substantially skewed account of what transpired, leaving out a high-quality deal of records.

It all comes right all the way down to disposing of context from what you preference to show. Propagandists regularly lease this tactic to spread their message.

It’s an vintage story of a partially advised truth.

Sincere disagreements and constructive grievance are normally desired. However, complaint want to originate from a properly-founded clinical attitude in choice to an emotional response.

You've without a doubt heard the announcing, "I might not permit everybody hypnotize me."What precisely are they announcing, and what does hypnosis suggest for someone like that?

For them, hypnosis is similar to a "magic spell" that induces regular helplessness and reliance on the hypnotist.

We have already talked about how this fake concept can rise up due to the manner hypnosis is normally blended with ordinary fictional narratives.

In cutting-edge day, the hypnotic country denotes a moment even as the conscious thoughts is absent. They fear that they'll display screen the darker aspect of themselves compulsively, admit their animosity, or display facts they might in no way willingly proportion with everyone.

This is the actual chance they understand with hypnosis. They attack it to guard themselves in the direction of it.

It's corresponding to the fervent, violent, and charismatic attacks to relieve his private guilt approximately the fact that he is surely attracted to vice.

Although it could take many particular workplace paintings, worry of hypnosis is essentially the priority of sharing one's real feelings.

For example, an worker who become at odds along with his business enterprise and who he despises may also in no way agree to be hypnotized although the possibility arose.

He is probably scared of pronouncing or doing a little issue that could jeopardize his recognition.

For him, hypnosis might be "risky" because of the truth he wouldn’t need to take the risk.

In fact, in spite of the reality that, this man or woman might be taking a danger. The hypnotic united states of america isn't always a time for confession. The problem is continuously aware of his words.

The situation informs the hypnotist if he is unwilling to answer any greater questions.

If the hypnotist persevered on this way, the issue may additionally spoil unfastened from the hypnotic kingdom.

This poses a risk to a person's protection. In fact, the hypnotic state is a hyper acute 2nd of excessive attention for the undertaking. Additionally, the priority does not, inner the right revel in of the word, constitute a shut eye or a rustic of nirvana.

Despite being in a modified state of awareness, his faculties and reasoning live intact.

The approach of inducing hypnosis sincerely produces a heightened usa of suggestibility.

When the general public and the clinical community understand the real nature of hypnosis, we can be capable of use this power with greater popularity.

It is a slow schooling manner however it's going to in the end development. In the save you, I assume the quality hazard that a person who fears hypnosis faces comes from any subjective issues he can also moreover have approximately his very own emotional participation in the hypnotic approach.

Naturally, surely absolutely everyone utilising hypnosis to reduce ache ought to talk with their circle of relatives medical scientific medical doctor.

Pain is nature's method of telling us that there may be a hassle with the organism. It would be foolish to mean that a pain within the belly will leave at the same time as, in fact, this could mean the need for an appendix manner. Regarding persistent migraine headaches, the same can be said.

It is important to check that the headache isn't a sign of a cancerous tumor or some unique pathological state of affairs. It might be exciting to understand that terminal maximum cancers patients are currently receiving hypnosis to help with their ache.

Currently, hypnosis is used by numerous thousand dentists country wide. The Journal of the American Society of Psychosomatic Dentistry is a quarterly magazine posted through this organization, which has installed its very very own society.

Chapter 10: Is Hypnosis the Answer?

A phrase of caution in opposition to 3 attitudes which have received traction and are aptly confirmed inside the medical discipline might be prudent. Direct idea is illegal on this regard.

One typically compelled adage is in no way disposing of the symptom till the motive is known.

Given that a large part of clinical practice consists of direct symptom removal and that simplest a small amount of idea goes into making an obvious

Another drastically ordinary rule is that on the way to efficiently address symptom complexes, the subconscious historical past want not constantly be made aware of.

This statement will become an entire lot less credible even as low-cost and thoughtful interest of the big characteristic of the subconscious in every day residing and functioning is given.

I have to flow into greater element about each of those statements because of the fact they continuously come up inside the minds of people who are searching out hypnotic assist.

The first aspect that includes thoughts is that each one of the religious recovery stated inside the Bible at once deal with signs and symptoms and signs.

Direct symptom removal is some different place wherein non secular devotees' visits to hallowed shrines offer treatment plans.

I actually have now not but heard all and sundry criticize spiritual leaders for being dealt with on this manner or denounce non secular shrines. These healing are credited to the supernatural or said as evidence of the effectiveness of religion.

Nothing is ever completed inside the ones situations to assist the character get better or realize the character of the subconscious methods that induced his trouble.

It is inadequate to put in writing off non secular recuperation with the phrase "it isn't always clinical.

If a technique is effective, then it's miles medical. If it does now not help the person that is on the lookout for assistance, it is useless.

We must widely known that not all and sundry responds nicely to the identical mental interventions.

This is without troubles seen in the intense example: An Aboriginal person experiencing mental troubles maximum without a doubt could now not be a appropriate candidate for psychoanalysis as we currently apprehend it.

Without a doubt, a witch scientific doctor may additionally need to help him loads greater genuinely.

It additionally makes enjoy that any knowledgeable Westerner ought to now not be swayed by using manner of a tribal medicine guy's incantations.

As we look at in addition, we find out that there are various psychotherapy colleges and strategies for resolving emotional problems in humans.

However, the remedy rate is more or much less the identical for they all. I think we need to renowned that there isn't a single particular, rational, medical answer.

As extended because of the fact the favored final outcomes is attained, I assume the technique have become clinical sufficient to meet anyone's wishes.

All treatment plans cause to help the affected man or woman in freeing themselves from any emotional issues that may be bothering them.

Some readers might also additionally furthermore find this technique to be an oversimplification of a completely complicated trouble, however I obtain as proper with it's time for us to have a practical components freed from technical jargon.

All too often, failures had been glibly defined away with convoluted technical terms and theories.

Rather than focusing maximum of the time on looking for to decide out why the patient isn't always feeling nicely, I suppose we need to be placing an growing quantity of emphasis on steps to help the affected individual enjoy better. Naturally, that is symptom removal over again.

I would like to draw interest to a charming reality about biblical healers. Since the healer's recognition preceded him in every state, he changed into capable of heal the sick. He did, however, find out no religion and later no remedy in locations wherein his reputation as a healer end up both unknown or discredited.

It is proper that via placing a robust emphasis on sound judgment and requirements, it has assisted in putting a prevent to unbridled creativity and careless paintings practices.

However, the overemphasis on objectivity and the rigidly single necessities of pleasant techniques have

I assume the majority of humans recognize how they came to have their cutting-edge problems quite properly. I've yet to satisfy the person that complains that he could no longer apprehend why he cannot carry out to his complete capacity in a particular state of affairs.

Practically talking, few humans have the time or resources to analyze the trouble's unconscious roots.

The objection to the excessive fee of treatment are valid and ought to now not be overlooked lightly. Individuals with emotional problems normally revel in financial setbacks as well.

Who will assist those people? There are not many locations throughout the country in which human beings can get low-price, expert intellectual health care. Exists assist of this kind to your close by network?

Only in instances wherein an character turns into destitute does the u . S . Offer its help. However, the road decrease decrease back to sound emotional fitness is presently an extended and difficult one.

Approximately 10 million copies of two hundred excellent pamphlets overlaying numerous factors of intellectual fitness are distributed through the National Association for Mental Health and its branches.

Our dependable call of the item is "Mental Health Education: A Critique." Ernest

Hangman's feature "Who's Normal? "In the August eight, 1960 trouble of Life includes a completely profitable article approximately this convention.

How approximately psychoanalysis and psychiatry? This is an unrelated hassle. Psychotherapy has helped plenty of sad and people, but now not absolutely everyone who has attempted it has determined achievement.

In truth, all of the highbrow fitness booklets, which characteristic an epilogue to the self-assist strategies they promote, give up by way of way of advising the reader to are in search of professional assist if their issues are severe sufficient.

However, the critics at Cornell pointed to data that, in their opinion, confirmed that receiving psychiatric remedy is as far flung for the standard man or woman as going to the moon.

Most readers of this book, I anticipate, are aware about the under staffing of nation hospitals. And incapable of giving the mentally unwell the care they want.

The govt director of the National Mental Health Committee, Mike German, has authored a groundbreaking document in this real subject matter titled Every Other Bed.

In addition to the greater giant untold human struggling that can be translated into bucks, intellectual contamination charges the usa of the united states 2.Five billion dollars every year.

The ebook tells the horrifying tale of the way we allowed this to occur, how we hold to permit it to happen, and the way little the overall public, further to the clinical and mental professions, are doing to address this abhorrent state of affairs.

It's time to reevaluate the adages that kingdom that a symptom can not be cured until the underlying reason is diagnosed and that signs and symptoms need to be introduced to mild that allows you to understand their unconscious origins.

There had been a number of notable-selling books these days that complex in this equal subject. Does it feature? Yes, it is on the equal time as used as it should be.

You may be tremendous that this non secular psychology has been criticized. The critique is that the unconscious warfare remains unresolved and that the important reasons of the difficulty are in no manner addressed.

It's the identical argument made over and over. What approximately the those who have been assisted? They seem to have finished tremendous topics, are in fee of lives, and feature adjusted in reality all and sundry else.

Once infused with this uplifting spirit of nicely-being, it definitely permeates each degree in their relationships. The best cause for the dearth of complaint is that the ones corporations' religious ideals embody this form of psychotherapy, and criticizing another person's religion renders the critic's whole worldview insupportable.

I wholeheartedly help these groups because I might as an alternative have a faith that usually emphasizes life's first-rate additives and the concept t How to Attain Self-Hypnosis h How to Attain Self-Hypnosis at "lifestyles may be beautiful" if one puts their religion in God and adopts an advantageous outlook.

It is surely most suitable to the merciless ideologies of its opponents or the difficult religions that emphasize punishment. Consider the emotions of guilt related to the latter.

Nobody can maintain such an remarkable cult. Naturally, if we suggest to non secular, brilliant-wondering people that they will be education self-hypnosis, they will vehemently dispute and argue the point.

As our primary subject is mental hygiene in desire to prevailing a debate, it is satisfactory to depart the hassle as it stands.

The thing to preserve in thoughts is that, as long as an character believes that this technique is the great manner to meet his dreams and as long as nobody is harmed thru his conviction, I expect he want to paste to it. He need to not allow individuals who use one-of-a-kind semantic phrases to discuss damage it.

I want to speak approximately one greater commonplace instance that relates to the 2 essential mind that we were speakme approximately. It is an example of the severa human beings who have conquer degree fright with the aid of enrolling in public speaking courses.

The majority of the time, the character in query hasn't had many opportunities to speak in public.

This makes him experience as even though he may also say the incorrect element or neglect what he have turn out to be going to mention.

This anxiety can motive any situation or obstacle that he fears. What's the restoration? Psychoanalysis, for positive, isn't the manner to find out why he operates the manner he does. This is one technique you may take, but it is now not the most effective, for my part.

It's similar to asking, "What can I do that's right?" instead of, "What am I doing it without a doubt is incorrect?" Enrolling in a path of education to benefit realistic revel in and exercising in public speakme techniques is the most useful method.

Before going any further, I anticipate it's far critical to make smooth that I'm now not sincerely criticizing the ideals of different sincere and devoted people going for walks within the location of intellectual hygiene. It is mostly a proper concept to rethink our present day positions on any given hassle, regardless of how earnest or high-quality we may be that our moves are justified.

Sometimes, we're capable of emerge as so emotionally invested in our ideals that we discover it tough to in fact be given grievance and react emotionally to ideas or interpretations that defy motive.

So what are the answers to intellectual health troubles? No unmarried solution exists. It's a very complex situation. A lot of labor wants to cross into developing and enforcing the many promising medicinal tablets and treatments which have the capability to significantly beautify intellectual fitness.

The important trouble will continually be looking to recognize human behavior and offering powerful remedies for those in need. What is the approach for that? I think hypnosis can assist with a part of the solution.

Hypos is glaringly contraindicated in lots of emotional problems due to the individual of the issue. It is critical to address super emotional issues on a conscious stage first. After that, hypnosis may be useful in engaging in the final goal.

Chapter 11: How Does Self Hypnosis Work?

You may probably even take a superstar's inclinations to acquire the characteristics you desire. If this isn't always feasible, create a personality that embodies everything you want to be.

Imagine you shifting, talking, and attractive in every day sports. Continue to reinforce this image with the critical intellectual sports activities.

It may not take lengthy for those mind to translate into the self-confident feelings you choice. You will surely integrate those images into your conscious persona as you continue to achieve this.

By the manner, undertaking the hypnotic usa of the usa itself can be finished with the equal machine. During your first attempts, you visualize yourself falling right into a nation of hypnosis. This ultimately creates the vital situations for a conditioned response and a powerful emotional response.

With this approach, the affected individual is usually recommended to "form a photo" in his thoughts whilst in a country of slight hypnosis, following the identity of the trouble's root purpose and as a thing of his re-schooling.

Numerous conditions are proposed, which incorporates ones that the affected character may additionally stumble upon in actual existence. He is knowledgeable to look himself in every one "as in real existence generally succeeding.

For example, the speaker can be requested to describe how snug and comfortable they sense at the same time as speaking to others.

Along with instructions at the way to create the ones success snap shots for him, the affected character is also reminded that he will best be capable of see himself as a fulfillment, that is what he desires to be. It does not take lengthy for the affected individual to demonstrate the benefits of his private 3-d movie shows because of the reality the photographs elicit the proper feelings.

After training this technique to college college students, plenty of them have asked, "Is that each one there can be to it? It seems so easy.

Of route, there can be more to it than that the person has to in fact do what they may be instructed. One of the hard factors of this shape of software is this. Let me list a number of the issues I've had even as trying to teach self-hypnosis.

As previously stated, one of the disturbing conditions is that the technique seems overly uncomplicated. Students begin to doubt.

They believes that so that you can get consequences, it must be extra difficult and involved. People need to, I bet, understand something that top notch comes after a tough war.

This technique does no longer include this. Naturally, I'm not pronouncing that if someone uses this approach, his problems will magically depart and his existence becomes happier than it end up earlier than.

We've been socialized to remember that a few trouble profitable can best be executed through tough, protracted war.

A critical idea of the American way of existence is that. We've grown acquainted with the idea that fear and warfare are inevitable in existence and that overcoming great portions of them is needed to attain any corporation.

I can first-class strain that all you want to acquire effects is the information on this e-book.

If you strive this system for a brief at the same time as and do no longer see any most important effects, you have to live with it and now not give up. This leads us to a extra element.

A lot of humans expect instant results after they begin using self-hypnosis. When they do now not gain the expected results proper away, they want to apprehend "what is wrong.

My commonplace response is that "not some element is incorrect" and that each one they want to do is hold following the commands constantly.

Of course, learning the fundamentals might now not make someone a outstanding typist, musician, actor, or athlete. It requires time to end up gifted.

I promise that everybody who makes use of and places this approach to use will find blessings from it.

A project in addressing any trouble is directing pragmatism and melancholy. The advice that you supply yourself can encompass posthypnotic corrective measures. But I count on we moreover need to cope with them on a aware diploma.

No matter how prolonged your issues had been, you want to have confidence that you can overcome them. You gets the self-assist you need in case you're willing to paintings with self-hypnosis always.

You also can moreover from time to time expect a setback in your improvement, however this must not deter you from completing your goal in the end. List the accomplishments up to now.

If you feel "downed" due to the fact you have been hoping for faster and further dramatic results, preserve in thoughts that many folks that conflict with emotions revel in comparable feelings. Don’t neglect about how lengthy the hassle has been there.

You have in reality tried opportunity strategies and gave up at the same time as you didn't see the favored effects. You abandoned the belief and observed yourself returned on the begin.

Make a aware choice to paintings with unwavering morality further to a perseverance that allows you to no longer waver due to the truth your chosen intention will now not constantly be achieved.

I am aware about hypnotherapy that produces steady, splendid outcomes with out boundaries or sporadic setbacks.

Despite setbacks alongside the way, fulfillment is finished because of the fact the very last route has been carefully taken into consideration and laid out.

Finally, self-hypnosis might be powerful because of the truth you are usually schooling your unconscious to answer in a advantageous, powerful manner.

It is inevitable that the program will sooner or later grow to be automatic. When it does, you may find out which you are experiencing the desired feelings and the use of self hypnosis to accomplish the desires you got right down to advantage. In truth, you domesticate the emotions you choice.

Skeptics won't advantage from hypnosis.

These people often come into my workplace asking for help. He informs me that both his partner or his family medical doctor believes he must sign on in myself hypnosis direction.

I ask him if he thinks the route can be beneficial to him. If, after discussing the benefits of hypnosis with him in detail, he no matter the truth that would no longer seem geared up for the path, and if his reaction is poor, I ought to suggest finding a in reality one in all a kind way to address him.

The reason for this is that self-hypnosis clearly may not function as successfully as it'd otherwise except the man or woman is upbeat and captivated with it. The fine forces we preference to harness are restrained via manner of manner of the very nature of a skeptical mind-set.

Sometimes, people trying to find unquestionable evidence that hypnosis will gain them. Giving them the evidence and unequivocal assurance they call for isn't possible.

These same humans do no longer, however, want validation from their medical docs. Nobody can promise success. I do take a look at, although, that persistent and clever use of self-hypnosis can help guide the healing technique.

It is frequently essential to take a metaphysical approach in area of a scientific one. It's about seeking to meet the wishes of the affected individual. Occasionally, letting the affected person attend a class on self-hypnosis is useful.

Often, it takes clearly conversation and identification with considered one of a type self-hypnotists to alter his thoughts-set. Particularly whilst one or more college

college college students record experiencing full-size changes,

Because we are capable of acclimate ourselves to some of stimuli, self-hypnosis is powerful. We alter each consciously and unconsciously to quite some sports activities activities. Anxiety is the surrender result of a conditioning way that could or won't have been conscious. During self-hypnosis, the individual intentionally works to decorate and located into practice his very very personal innate capabilities.

When those goals are completed, emotions of self-warranty, rest, self manage, and nicely being check.

Hypnosis additionally makes use of a normal intellectual approach. Placebos, as all of us recognize, function remarkably in loads of situations.

An inactive substance or schooling, administered to pleasure or gratify a affected individual, drastically applied in managed studies to decide the overall performance of medicinal substances," is how the dictionary defines a placebo.

Several well-done studies have examined that humans get comparable consequences even as taking a actual remedy that turned into prescribed or a placebo, which they mistakenly take delivery of as actual with to be the medicine. Antihistamine checks were accomplished so as to save you colds numerous years inside the past. The outcomes remained consistent.

What reasons the placebo to feature in truth further to the real remedy is what interests us. It makes revel in that a highbrow response devices off a chain reaction that in the long run results in a physiological response. The patient, no longer know-how what's taking region, publicizes, Ive in no way felt so proper in my existence.

However, this may now not have happened if he hadn't believed he become taking the splendid new remedy.

A latest scientific look at by the use of one of the pinnacle pharmaceutical companies positioned that the affected person's religion inside the prescribing clinical medical physician money owed for one-0.33 of the effectiveness of any medicine.

The affected person's be given as real with inside the clinical health practitioner and the placebo impact, I'm positive, are elements that make contributions to the effectiveness of medicines that don't encompass a caution.

We are cognizant of this statistics. Our issues relate to the way to use this subconscious technique for advantageous purposes. The solution lies interior you. Induction

As we've got defined, visible imagery is a way applied in self-hypnosis. Although there are numerous names for this, we're capable of in reality call it visible imagery for the features of this speak.

This method consists of one of the keys to engaging in your desired goals. Numerous famous books have been written the use of this technique as a foundation for fulfillment.

The majority of the books in this subject are directed thru way of Dr. Emile Coupe's e-book, Self Mastery through Conscious Auto-Suggestion. The greater mature readers of this ebook have probable heard of his well-known saying, which I will reiterate with emphasis."Day through way of daylight hours very way is getting better and better."Every this type of books always makes connection with the biblical Old Testament of the Bible "As a man thicket in his coronary coronary coronary heart, souse

As you probable can infer, we are not conjecturing approximately an outstanding new locating. The approach is as old as humanity and the choice for a brighter future.

If the hassle is one in each of material wealth, all books that rent the visible-imagery method recommend you to create a concise highbrow picture of the fabric goods you preference to attain. Paint a clean image of the individual you need to be so as to enhance yourself.

You are commonly knowledgeable to do that with as few distractions as feasible at the equal time as in a relaxed or contemplative united states.

Again, are they not in reality discussing the unconscious mind?

I disagree with any sensible approach for selling emotional development, but I do remember that we are more and more attractive with semantics the means of phrases. Self-hypnosis is the quickest route to the subconscious. You can intentionally direct tips for your subconscious mind at the same time as you are in this self-hypnotic United States of America.

Chapter 12: the Self Hypnotic State

You will see that the commands on a way to accumulate self-hypnosis come in advance than this bankruptcy. This is finished to allay any fears you could have approximately the solution to the question,

If I'm hypnotized, how do I awaken myself?" It is vital to realize that, regardless of being hypnotized, you continue to have manipulate over your frame, are aware about your surroundings and what is taking place round you, are able to assume definitely, and can without problems rouse yourself.

Saying or thinking the phrases "I shall now open my eyes and wake up feeling brilliant" is all that is required. Another preference is to set a depend for you, inclusive of "As I rely to five, I'll open my eyes and awaken feeling wonderfully well and refreshed. One, , three, 4, 5.

It is important to hold in thoughts that regardless of the truth that we time period the hypnotic united states of america of america sleep" at instances, we aren't speaking of actual sleep. This explains a large a part of the confusion.

If I'm asleep, how can I awaken myself?" the person wonders. This might be the case if the task modified into in reality unconscious. In reality, the problem is at a completely unique or expanded diploma of recognition.

While in self-hypnosis, he seems passive on the outdoor, however he's actually as a substitute aware.

When inside the self-hypnotic state, the man or woman intentionally shows matters to himself. This demonstrates that he is aware and that, with the proper recommendation, he can awaken himself.

Every now after which, the hassle nods off at the same time as a laugh or making guidelines to him in case you want to enter the perfect mental country. In this case, the scenario will surely wake up in the end.

The difficulty may also wake up inside the morning feeling rested if he practices hypnosis at his everyday time of falling asleep in mattress.

Prior to starting to offer recovery suggestions to yourself, you could offer your self the following suggestions, in order to indicate how lengthy you can paintings with self-hypnosis:

I'm going to exercising self-hypnosis for fifteen minutes. When that component includes an stop, I'll open my eyes and awaken feeling noticeably properly, alert, and confident.

Happy and upbeat. My eyes will open and I'll sense renewed. I'll be capable of awaken right away, live completely alert, and react efficiently in the event of any outside risk."

You'll see that those pointers account for the functionality for sports like fires and different risks that would endanger the man or woman. These are legitimate worries that the majority of individuals who strive self-hypnosis have. You can also software an alarm clock to wake you at a particular time.

Assume for the instant the if you want to wake yourself up, you advised to your self that you open your eyes and be simply huge extensive wakeful at 5. You count number range to five, but you can't appear to open your eyes for a few difficulty reason.

Firstly, please do not worry. Stay calm and repeat the advice to yourself, telling your self that you may real be capable of open your eyes without problems and feel OK on the trouble of 0.

I want the idea of now not being able to wake up hasn't scared you away. I simplest deliver this up to familiarize you with the technique. In reality, deny pan Attain Self-Hypnosis to state of no activity isn't a common trouble. I need to attract hobby to a vital fact.

Never once have I had a customer who come to be self-hypnotizing or working inside the route of inform me that he had even the slightest trouble waking up from the hypnotic nation.

People have advised me they have got have a look at or heard of a case wherein the problem slept for a number of days due to the reality the hypnotist become no longer able to loose them from the hypnotic country.

Not a unmarried story might be written down. Stage hypnotists used to vicinity a subject to sleep for numerous days in a shop window for publicity functions.

However, this have come to be voluntary, so it must no longer be careworn with what we're speakme approximately.

It is especially uncommon for me to art work with subjects who proved now not capable of fail to awaken at a predetermined recollect, however I honestly have had this revel in. Usually, what I discover is that the state of affairs is so comfortable that he virtually does now not want to awaken for worry of dropping this incredible feeling.

Chapter 13: How to Attain Self Hypnosis

Let's start with the idea that self hypnosis is technological information that everybody can look at and workout to a degree. We will presume that you have given cautious attention to what you desire to acquire. You have superior practical goals for remedy and self-development via self evaluation.

The acquisition of the hypnotic kingdom is the very last phase, consistent with se.

Before I offer you with the specific commands, allow me cope with a not unusual query that comes up even as teaching university students self-hypnosis. It's: Are recommendations that I supply myself as powerful as those you could provide me inhaler hypnosis?

Although it makes revel in to consider that the hypnotist's tips is probably greater beneficial than the difficulty's personal, each are further precious on an intrinsic diploma.

Recall that every one kinds of hypnosis are definitely styles of hypnosis for oneself, and that every one hetero suggestions are in reality transposed into kinds of self-tips.

The problem will automatically and unconsciously rephrase the statement from this 2d, I will experience very confident in all situations in lifestyles if the hypnotist strongly indicates, From this second, you'll experience very assured in all existence conditions.

Generally, the concern repeats all tips, every mentally or out loud, substituting the pronoun I for your.

Being hypnotized and receiving a posthypnotic idea that you can prompt a hypnotic kingdom in your self at any time you pick out out is the high-quality and fastest approach of analyzing self hypnosis.

The hypnotist does now not need to be an expert. Anyone who's familiar with the fundamentals of hypnosis can perform this. But assume you need to discover ways to hypnotize yourself and are unable to get assistance.

If you comprehend the instructions and consciously take a look at them, you may succeed in accomplishing your intention.

Take a seat in an smooth chair, or lie lower back on a bed or couch. Next, pick out out a place on the ceiling wherein you want to popularity your gaze, ideally someplace within the returned of you in which eye pressure or fatigue can also want to usually rise up.

Breathe deeply and really slowly now. Repeat mentally the terms "sleep" as you inhale and "deep sleep" as you completes this.

Repeat this for several minutes in an uneventful manner, or till you begin to experience sleepy. Then, tell your self that your eyelids are getting droopy and fatigued. Using this method, the purpose is to acquire eye closure. You want to get to the factor in which it hurts to open your eyes.

At the instant your eyes close to, reputedly in your very very own initiative, you have got correctly completed the number one level of self hypnosis.

You can tell your self such things as, "My eyelids have become absolutely heavy and tired over and over. My eyes have grow to be in reality moist. My eyelids are final. I actually need to close my eyes.

When I close my eyes, I'll drift off to a legitimate-soothing, deep sleep. Even in a deeply hypnotized u . S ., I can be aware of my surroundings and in a position to speak with my unconscious thoughts through posthypnotic suggestions.

Repeating affirmations alongside those equal lines will intensify these feelings while your eyelids truely get heavy or your eyes start to water.

This is called "the feed-once more method," and it serves to decorate the modern-day scenario. In this way, the actual ultimate of the eyes and the success of the hypnotic state are accelerated.

Assume for the immediate that while you follow this way, not something seems to expose up. Practice it again and again till you're able to advantage an eye fixed constant closure.

Over time, you'll be in a function to perform this in a relatively brief quantity of time.

You need to apply the method in fact given as frequently as possible on the equal time as you're falling asleep at night time time. With the lights out, you're mendacity in mattress. Select an opening for your thoughts this is every above and in the returned of your eyes to alleviate any pressure in your eye muscle mass.

Now begin telling your self matters likes "your eyelids have come to be heavy," and lots of others.

The hints you are making to your self throughout this time are what motive self-hypnosis to be so powerful because of the truth they seep into your unconscious as you skip from focus to subconscious cesspits similar to telling your self to rise up at a selected time each morning.

Your unconscious is made aware of the notion, which then reasons you to awaken consciously.

By the usage of this technique, you can provide yourself placed up-hypnotic recommendations that the subsequent time you exercise self hypnosis, you will input a deeper, sounder hypnotic state on the rely of 3, in addition to dynamic, outstanding tips at this thing.

Additionally, you strain that your eyelids will routinely near after 5 mins of rest.

And then rely backwards to a few. The use of the sleep period will beautify this conditioning system.

During this time, the guidelines will in all likelihood act subconsciously, accelerating your success of the high fine dreams and the self hypnotic intention that you set for your self.

The following suggestions will assist you input a deeper hypnotic us of a as quickly as you have acquired eye closure:

As I depend to 3, I shall skip deeper and deeper right into a profound, hypnotic state." I'm going to be conscious that my degree of relaxation will increase as I depend to three. I'm going to go into a deep, hypnotic sleep as speedy as I count to 3.

You again and again repeat the ones hints, really making an try to revel in extra snug, calmer, and further cushty. In doing so, you adopt the tendencies of a profoundly hypnotized problem.

Learning self-hypnosis can be difficult in issue due to the fact the practitioner is trying to result in a mental state for which he has no preceding experience. You can reply as it should be if I say,

Act happy or Act unhappy sink you may at once apprehend the reaction primarily based totally to your past tales.

It is crucial that you behave in a manner that you might likely anticipate approving buddies hypnosis if you have in no way visible someone in the u . S . Of even in times of a trance degree and I assist you to recognize to act as despite the fact that you've got been hypnotized.

You need to obviously count on the trends you had noticed in case you had simply witnessed a person hypnotized. Either one may do this knowingly or unknowingly.

The hypnotic United States is defined through a few as a nation of "whole rest. Many experience "detachment," at the equal time as others revel in "disassociation," feeling as despite the fact that their complete being is excellent a idea.

A "floating" or "drifting" sensation is experienced by means of manner of using a few, who look at it to mendacity on thick clouds. Some enjoy a thick, comfy, "sinking" sensation. Others experience "peace and calmness."Many people describe the hypnotic state as being just like the kingdom proper before falling asleep or as daydreaming, and that they've comparable reports.

www.ingramcontent.com/pod-product-compliance
Lightning Source LLC
Chambersburg PA
CBHW051727050625
27761CB00039B/448
9781775113997